Death and Decision

AAAS Selected Symposia Series

Published by Westview Press
5500 Central Avenue, Boulder, Colorado

for the

American Association for the Advancement of Science
1776 Massachusetts Ave., N.W., Washington, D.C.

Death and Decision

Edited by
Ernan Mc Mullin

AAAS Selected Symposium 18

AAAS Selected Symposia Series

Published in 1978 in the United States of America by

  Westview Press, Inc.
  5500 Central Avenue
  Boulder, Colorado 80301
  Frederick A. Praeger, Publisher and Editorial Director

Library of Congress Number: 77-18444
ISBN: 0-89158-152-9

Printed and bound in the United States of America

About the Book

Advances in technology have enabled the medical profession to keep people alive long after the normal possibilities of human living--and even of consciousness itself--have ceased. The Karen Quinlan case has focused public attention on the painful decision faced by those involved in such instances and on the intractability of the moral, medical, legal, and economic issues involved. These issues are not new; indeed, such problems are as old as death itself. But the burden laid on us by our own science, and by our own altered family structures, appears to be of a new order. It raises issues that intimately affect the quality of life in our society and that require new approaches. The issues discussed in this book demand the sensitive attention of doctors, theologians, philosophers, social workers, lawyers--of all those, in short, whose work brings them in contact with the kind of decision the voluntary termination of life represents.

Contents

Foreword

The *AAAS Selected Symposia Series* was begun in 1977 to
provide a means for more permanently recording and more
widely disseminating some of the valuable material which is
discussed at the AAAS Annual National Meetings. The volumes
in this *Series* are based on symposia held at the Meetings
which address topics of current and continuing significance,
both within and among the sciences, and in the areas in which
science and technology impact on public policy. The *Series*
format is designed to provide for rapid dissemination of information, so the papers are not typeset but are reproduced
directly from the camera copy submitted by the authors, without copy editing. The papers are reviewed and edited by
the symposia organizers who then become the editors of the
various volumes. Most papers published in this *Series* are
original contributions which have not been previously published, although in some cases additional papers from other
sources have been added by an editor to provide a more com-
prehensive view of a particular topic. Symposia may be reports of new research or reviews of established work, particularly work of an interdisciplinary nature, since the AAAS
Annual Meeting typically embraces the full range of the
sciences and their societal implications.

WILLIAM D. CAREY
Executive Officer
American Association for
the Advancement of Science

About the Editor and Authors

Ernan Mc Mullin is professor of philosophy at the University of Notre Dame. The author of numerous articles on the history and theory of the scientific method, he is concerned with questions raised by the knowledge-claims of science and other areas of human concern (history, art, theology). He is the author of Galileo, Man of Science *(1967) and the editor of* The Concept of Matter in Modern Philosophy *(Notre Dame, 1963). His most recent work is a study of the epistomological structures of clinical judgement in medicine.*

Eric J. Cassell is a clinical professor in the Department of Public Health, Cornell University Medical College. He has published numerous papers on the use of language in medicine and on the philosophy of clinical practice, including "Language as a Tool in Medicine" (with L. Skopek in Journal of Medical Education, Vol. 52, *March, 1977). He is also the author of* The Healer's Art *(Lippincott, 1976).*

H. Tristram Engelhardt, Jr., is the Rosemary Kennedy Professor of Philosophy of Medicine, Kennedy Institute, Center for Bioethics, Georgetown University, Washington, DC. His area of concern is the philosophy of medicine and medical ethics, and he is an associate editor of the Journal of Medicine and Philosophy. *He is the author of* Mind-Body: A Categorial Relation *(The Hague, Martinus Nighoff, 1973).*

Philippa Ruth Foot, now a professor of philosophy at UCLA, was senior research fellow and tutor at Somerville College, Oxford University, England. A Fellow of the British Academy, she is the editor of Theories of Ethics *(Oxford University Press, 1967) and has published articles and reviews in both scholarly and popular journals. A collection of her essays,* Virtues and Vices and Other Essays in Moral Philosophy *is forthcoming (Blackwell's, in press).*

*Alasdair MacIntyre is University Professor of philosophy
and political science in the Political Science, Sociology,
Philosophy and University Professors' Program, Boston University. His areas of specialization are moral philosophy,
history and sociology of moral change, and medical ethics,
and his recent publications are in the area of values and
medical practice.*

*William F. May is professor and chairman of the Depart-
ment of Religious Studies, Indiana University, Bloomington.
He has published numerous articles and essays on theology
and medical ethics in* The Hastings Center Report, Social
Research, *the* Journal of the American Academy of Religion,
and in various other anthologies.

*E. Mansell Pattison is professor and vice-chairman of
the Department of Psychiatry and Human Behavior, University
of California, Irvine. Specializing in social psychiatry,
he is the author of several books, most recently* The Experience of Dying *(Prentice-Hall, 1976). He has also published
numerous research and clinical papers in the field of
thanatology, including "Help in the Dying Process,"* (American
Handbook of Psychiatry; *Basic, 1974).*

*Leslie S. Rothenberg is acting professor of law at
Loyola University School of Law, California. He is interested in the legal aspects of the "right to die" and is author
of* Law, Medicine and Religion: The Karen Quinlan Case *(to be
published). He participated in formulation of guidelines
for the use of the "Directive to Physicians" to discontinue
life-sustaining treatment in terminal illnesses, as recently
authorized by law in California, the first state to pass
such a statute.*

*Thomas C. Schelling is the Lucius N. Littauer Professor
of Political Economy, John F. Kennedy School of Government,
Harvard University. His special concerns are the processes
of conflict, strategy, and collective decision. He is the
author of* The Strategy of Conflict *(Harvard University Press,
1960), "The Life You Save May Be Your Own" (in Samuel Chase
[Ed.],* Problems in Public Expenditure Analysis; *Brookings
Institution, 1968), and "On Choosing Our Children's Genes"
(in Mack Lipkin, Jr. and Peter T. Rowley,* Genetic Responsibility, *Plenum Press, 1974).*

Death and Decision

Introduction

Ernan Mc Mullin

Death has never quite seemed to lie within the bounds
of human decision, as other episodes do. Of course, killing
has always gone on, and under certain circumstances has been
thought proper. The exacting of death as a punishment for
serious crime may be as old as man himself. Human sacrifice
and the exposing of unwanted children have been recurrent
features of the human story. And in our unending wars,
soldiers and civilians die by the hand of others; it is
regretted but nonetheless praised. But these are special
circumstances; in the normal course, man may not deprive
another of life, nor may he take responsibility for further-
ing his own death. Murder and suicide are wrong; even
carelessness that may hasten the death of another or of
oneself is seriously culpable.

In the Western tradition, our attitudes on these issues
have been shaped to a large extent by Christian theology,
and specifically by the doctrines of creation, resurrection,
and redemption. God is not merely a shaper of recalcitrant
matter; human life is not a punishment, nor an unending
sequence of unwanted recurrences. God is creator of all;
matter serves Him and time is his first creature, since it
is within time that His plan is to be realized. Life is His
making, and human life is the unique once-only-given
opportunity to become as like to Him as material restrictions allow. Death marks the end of becoming for the individual; at the moment of death, his life is irrevocably what
he has made it. But it is not the end in the sense of
cessation of being. It is the beginning of a new existence
with God, no longer bound by the limitations of time,
decision, and change. Life is thus God's first and greatest
gift; one owes it the reverence proper to such a gift. And
death is not a loss of this gift so much as its fulfilment,
the moment of self-gathering when all the strands of a life
fall finally into pattern and take on a definitive and

permanent reality.

Man's freedom is shadowed by man's weakness, his
ability to turn from God. It is also shadowed by suffering,
which is inescapably the lot of a finite creature of human
aspirations and human sensibilities. The Judaeo-Christian
tradition has always linked sin and suffering, has seen them
as somehow derivative from a genuine freedom on the part of
a creature to reject its Creator. The agonized death of
Christ on a cross led Christians further to see in his
sacrifice a form of redemption, a buying-back of fallen man,
a restoration to man of the possibilities meant for him.
Christ could have avoided suffering; that he did not, and
that his suffering took on the meaning it did, made of pain
and deprivation borne in the service of others a holy thing,
something from which even the most virtuous could not be
exempt.

It is important to recall the details of the Christian
story of life and death, if one is to understand the depth
of the present perplexities in regard to the proper limits
of our power to decide when a particular life should terminate. There are two quite different sorts of reason why
these perplexities have multiplied in recent decades.
Medical science has advanced enormously in its ability to
extend life. It has also altered the conditions under
which the seriously ill are cared for, removing them almost
entirely from ordinary human contact. Questions of a new
sort arise as to how it should employ its powers, as to
what its precise goals ought to be, as to whom its decision-
making should involve. Medical science cannot of itself
develop answers to such questions. And the resources of the
Christian moral tradition are not sufficient to provide the
kind of straightforward guidance that people seek in matters
 of such urgency. Distinctions that have helped in the past
(such as that between extraordinary and ordinary means, or
between killing and allowing to die) do not seem to meet the
new situations that arise in everyday hospital practice.

If developments in medical science and therapeutic
techniques were all that had to be considered, the problems
would not appear quite as intractable as they do. There
is another sort of change whose implications for complex new
moral issues of this kind are much more far-reaching. This
is the growing pluralism in Western society in regard to
moral and social norms generally. The Christian tradition
no longer commands universal adherence, and no other source
of moral authority (of the kind the Party claims to be in
the Second World) has taken its place. Liberal democracy
has often been alleged to rest on a utilitarian ethic, yet

a wide diversity of metaethical principles quite evidently informs moral controversy in Western countries. And the notion of 'utility' is in any event so broad as not to be of much help in decisions about termination of life. When moral problems arise, of a kind that the conventional wisdom of our society does not seem able to handle, there are no longer agreed principles to which one can turn, there is no authority that can propose courses of action with the likelihood of their general acceptance.

What makes this sort of uncertainty all the more serious is that the decision to end a life on medico-moral grounds almost always involves groups of people: a hospital staff, a family ... A single doctor, or the patient, or a guardian, may take primary responsibility, but others are almost inevitably implicated too. If agreement on the relevant values is lacking, the further difficulty arises of devising a plan of action that will be acceptable to all concerned, and of deciding on the hierarchy of responsibilities among those involved.

It may be helpful to separate five different medical contexts in which the question of deliberately terminating a life may arise. There are important differences between the moral issues raised in each case.

Case A: Abortion is probably the commonest sort of deliberate life-termination. It is still an illegal act in a great many countries, but is quite commonplace in others, like Japan. The law will often specify restrictions (e.g. the foetus must be no more than six months old; the grounds must be the physical health of the mother, or that the conception followed rape, or that the foetus is known to have a serious defect ...). Few defenders of abortion would allow the killing of newborn infants. So that the controversy tends to focus around two sorts of issue. First, is the foetus fully "human" ? Does it have the same rights as it would have once it leaves the womb ? If not, why not ? It is difficult to see why separation from the womb should make a basic difference to the "humanness" or the "personhood" of the infant organism. Is there perhaps an earlier stage at which this transition to "humanness" occurs, at the point when separate existence is in principle possible, for example ? Or when the nervous system first begins to form ? Efforts to define and defend such points of transition have not been notably successful. Once the fertilized ovum is implanted, its development to biological maturity is continuous. Discontinuity occurs only in its relationship to its mother, when it ceases (or could cease) to be dependent on her.

A second set of problems centers around the question of appropriate grounds. The strongest justifying reason would be that the presence of the foetus endangers the life of the mother. In such a case, can the foetus be treated as an "aggressor" ? Or is it rather that the mother's "personhood" balanced against that of the foetus, justifies the preference given her ? Suppose it is not the life of the mother but only her convenience that is at stake ? She may not wish a child at this time for economic or social or personal reasons, and did not intend one to be conceived. How strong a reason ought she have to be morally justified in deciding on abortion ? Does it make a difference if the conception was against her will ? If the foetus is not the fruit of a fully free affirmative act on both sides, does it forfeit its right to life ?

There are two morally simple and consistent positions here: one, that abortion under any circumstances is wrong, the other that abortion for any non-frivolous reason is permissible. The "in-between" range of positions is morally complex because relative weight is being given to the various reasons for aborting a foetus on the one hand, as well as to its degree of development on the other. A balance is reached between the gravity of the reason and the loss caused, somewhat as in wartime decisions to bomb areas where civilian casualties are inevitable. The assessment of relative weight of the factors concerned is extremely diffi- cult, and dangerously subject to rationalization. The moral issues here are the more indefinite but no less important ones of selfishness, of reverence for life, of taking responsibility for the consequences of action. They do not admit of hard-and-fast norms, but depend on the maturity of an informed faculty of moral judgement, on the ability to make a just balance.

Case B: Suppose the foetus has grave physical defects. Can it be killed for its own good ? This raises rather different issues, ones that can be more readily stated for the newborn. If a newborn baby is so deformed that it cannot live long anyway, may its life be shortened, say by not feeding it ? If it suffers from some handicap (Down's syndrome, thalido- mide induced limb-loss ...) that will notably lessen the quality of life later open to it, may efforts to keep it alive be less energetic than for a normal child ?

From a utilitarian standpoint, the answer to such questions is relatively simple to state. Since such children are usually a heavy burden on their family, on hospital resources, on society generally, the greatest good of the greatest number would seem to require their rapid

and painless termination. And, of course, the same might be
said for the insane, for habitual criminals, and for other
groups of socially unwanted citizens. But the traditions of
Western society have never condoned this kind of answer.
Reverence for life as the unique gift of God, respect and
care for the weak, have been (and still remain) deeply
ingrained, and have led to a very different response.

This response would begin by rejecting utilitarian
norms, specifically the notion that the convenience of a
group (family, hospital, society) can serve as sufficient
warrant for the death of an individual. That a newborn
spina bifida is difficult and expensive to care for, that a
mongoloid child can be an emotionally disastrous burden for
its parents, are not accepted as proper reasons for depriving
a child of life. Rather one must ask: what is good for the
child itself ? How is its welfare to be safeguarded ?

If the child is not (so far as one can tell) in serious
pain, its welfare would seem to demand that ordinary care be
given to it, just as to a normal child. If it is seriously
handicapped, so that it is already clear that it cannot live
a full human life, it should still be cared for and helped
to the fullest enjoyment of whatever level of life is
possible to it. That this imposes burdens on family and
society is undeniable, but (according to this second view)
such burdens are an inescapable part of what it is to be
human. A full-hearted acceptance of them is thus a sign
of true maturity.

If the child is in great pain, the case is not much
different from that of an adult (Case E below). Causing the
child additional pain (by not feeding it, for example) seems
particularly hard to justify. Distinctions between active
and passive euthanasia, between extraordinary and ordinary
therapeutic means, are often cited in such cases but seem
inadequate to justify the actual causing of pain. If a
decision has been made to hasten the child's death, whatever
its merits, it is at least arguable that it should be carried
out painlessly.

There are thus two quite different general sorts of
response to Case B, one utilitarian and community-oriented,
the other Christian in its Western roots and oriented to the
welfare of the individual and the protection of life. And
there are various modifications of both; one might, for
example, attach considerable weight to the "utility", understood as happiness, of the child in arriving at a utilitarian
assessment. Or one might note that the acceptance of responsibility for the weak has very great value ("utility") for a

family or a community. But such considerations do not
disguise the fact that Case B can mark a parting of the moral
ways, as the history of Nazi Germany unforgettably showed.

<u>Case C:</u> The kind of case which has had most notoriety lately
is that of the comatose patient being kept alive by means of
a sophisticated technology. The enormous publicity given
the Quinlan case in the U.S. made it appear more or less
the paradigm, despite the fact that it did have some rather
special features. What is distinctive about Case C is,
first, that the patient himself or herself cannot be directly
consulted, second, that the quality of even minimal human
living has been irreparably lost, and finally, that biological life is being sustained only by the use of special
means (machines, drugs ...). Each of these clauses raises
a host of difficulties.

If the patient cannot be consulted, who <u>is</u> to bear the
responsibility for life - termination in such a case ? The
doctor or the patient's family ? Or both in consultation ?
Where there is disagreement, which should prevail ? If the
patient has signified in advance what his or her wishes
would be in such an outcome, ought this be given primary
weight ? This last has become a matter of much concern since
the notion of a "living will" became popular some years ago.

A disturbing recent development in the U.S. is the
transfer of decision-making in such cases to the law courts.
The threat (sometimes real, sometimes imagined) of malpractice
suits has transformed the practice of American medicine in
the past decade; hardly anyone would say that this has been
for the overall benefit of either patient or doctor. It has
made doctors unwilling to take responsibility for decisive
action in grey areas, where a lawyer may later be able to
argue that sufficient grounds for the action cannot be shown.
The termination of life-support for a permanently comatose
patient is a grey area, not so much for the usual reason
that the family might afterwards choose to sue, as for the
reason that under U.S. law such an action can plausibly be
construed as a criminal offence, i.e. murder. In practice,
doctors are far less willing now to take responsibility for
discontinuance of life-support than they were, because of
the publicity given such cases and the real uncertainty
(which state legislatures and the Congress have done nothing
to remove) about the legal situation.

The second feature of Case C is that it should be known
that normal human functioning cannot be restored. But how
is this to be known ? Sometimes there is such a destruction
of brain tissue, for example, that doctors can be "morally

certain" that restoration is impossible, i.e. no cases are
known where restoration of function followed such destruction,
and there are theoretical reasons for arguing in this case
that mental functioning would be impossible in the absence
of the needed organic support. But quite often, no such
conviction can be reached. It is a matter of probability
only, with the likelihood of disagreement between the medical
experts. If there is any reasonable chance that mental
function may be restored, is one entitled to terminate ?
Suppose there is a high likelihood of permanent brain damage,
ought this alter one's treatment of the comatose patient ?
In particular, would it justify the termination of life-
support specifically to prevent such an outcome, i.e. recovery from the coma with highly impaired brain-functioning ?

This last question is not typical of Case C; what is
peculiar to this sort of case is that one cannot call upon
the good of the patient as a factor in the decision, as one
ordinarily can elsewhere. If the patient is permanently
comatose, he is not suffering, is not unhappy. The termination no longer matters, one way or the other, to the patient.
It matters now only to the community. One can argue that
the patient would not have wanted to survive in this attenuated, and no longer fully human, way. The patient may, in
fact, have indicated this in advance; if he did not, it is
not (experience has shown) so easy to prove a presumptive
intention. In any event, the decision will usually hinge
on the relative weight given in the community to such factors
as reverence for life (and the consequent unwillingness to
take steps to end life even where the minimal possibility of
properly human living no longer exists), pain caused to
family, economic cost, allocation of scarce medical
resources, and so on.

There is a similarity between Case A and Case C in that
the foetus has not yet attained full human functioning,
and the permanently comatose patient cannot have it restored;
in both cases, this has been held to justify relaxation of
the normal prohibition on killing of humans. There is, of
course, an important difference between the two cases. The
foetus is "potentially" human, in the sense that, given
normal environment and nurture, it will become fully human;
the comatose patient has been but is no longer fully human.
The respect and care given him are a testimony not of his
present humanity, but of the physical continuity of this
organism with a person who was in the fullest sense to be
esteemed and protected.

Christians will want to ask: but has the soul left the
body ? is this organism we see in the hospital bed still a
son of God, not yet returned to the Father ? This is a

peculiarly intractable question. If one adopts a soul-body
dualism of the Platonic kind   often favored in the Christian
tradition, involving a natural immortality of spirit or soul,
then the question becomes: does soul remain in an organism
which no longer can sustain any of the higher functioning
characteristic of soul ? The answer would seem to be: no,
but there would be no unanimity about this in the Greek
philosophical tradition. On the other hand, if one returns
to the Jewish beliefs that underlay the Christian doctrine
of resurrection, immortality is not an inevitable consequence
of a spirit-constituent of man, rather it is a gift or cove-
nant involving the whole person. What goes back to God is
not the spirit (to which the body would be rather awkwardly
joined later) but the person, in his life and achievement as
a free and responsible being. This would suggest that if
this conscious life and achievement is definitively ended,
the human being is no longer there; he has (according to the
Christian hope)returned to God who first set him out on
his voyage.

The third feature of Case C is that biological life is
being sustained only by special means, so that if one were
to discontinue these, it is presumed the patient would die.
Once again, the first difficulty is how to be sure of this
as the Quinlan case dramatically demonstrated. When after
the long legal battle the patient was disconnected from the
support-machinery, she survived, to the great surprise of
most of the physicians who had been consulted about her
state. The emphasis given this aspect of Case C is due in
the main to the distinction between "extraordinary" and
"ordinary" therapy, the traditional principle being that one
is not compelled to resort to the former.

It is difficult, however, to draw this distinction in
practice. On which side does penicillin lie ? Is it a
question of the expense or of the complexity or of the
novelty of the proposed therapy ? One could make the case
that virtually all therapy in the modern hospital is "extraordinary"; conversely, one could argue that, given our
resources, it is "ordinary". But leaving aside the difficulties in making this distinction work, it may be asked whether
it has the importance in Case C it has been assumed to have.
It would be fairly generally agreed that complex life-support
may be withdrawn from a permanently comatose patient at the
discretion of medical staff and family. But the central
feature of Case C is not the "extraordinary" therapy, it is
the permanence of the cessation of conscious functioning.
Even if the patient is able to live without the aid of
expensive and unevenly available technology, the substantive
question still remains: what sort of efforts ought to be

made to keep him or her alive ?

There is a natural repugnance to the denial of food to an organism needing it for survival. But there are always drugs needed to ward off the diseases such a patient is prone to. The doctor would seem to have some discretion about whether or not to administer these drugs, not because they are "extraordinary", but because it might be said that continuance of biological life is not obligatory. How would this differ from administering a painless lethal drug ?

There has been a great deal of debate about the distinction between killing and allowing to die, active and passive euthanasia. Without rehearsing the details of this debate, it may at least be noted that the moral responsibility for the outcome in such cases as we have been discussing may well be the same whether the intervention of the doctor be "active" or "passive". What differs is rather a matter of appropriateness, none the less important for being described by this weaker term. The doctor is understood to have the discretion whether or not to administer a healing drug. But the administering of what would be, in effect, a poison is not only not something he can be required by others to do, it is not even seemly for someone whose function in the community is to restore health. There is no reason why the <u>doctor</u> should be the one to intervene actively in this manner. Assuming that it were moral to terminate the life of a comatose patient in this way, one might better ask a representative of the family (or, for that matter, a judge, if one were involved) to be the agent.

Would the use of a poison ever in fact be allowable in such a case ? In terms of effectiveness, it might be no more lethal in its action than the withholding of penicillin from a comatose patient with penumonia. Why is it, then, that most people would reject one course and not the other? Of the reasons that might be cited, perhaps the most convincing is that we have a clear duty not to kill our fellow humans, except in very special circumstances such as self-defence. We do not have so clear a duty to provide them with the necessities of life; this would ordinarily be a matter of charity rather than justice. When faced with a comatose patient, we are inclined to transfer the same principles, even though the case is now a quite special one.

Furthermore, the reverence for life so basic to Western culture would make killing a more serious infringement than allowing to die, even though the responsibility for the outcome may be the same. The choice of means makes a difference in terms of the attitude signified. Any weake-

ning in the inviolability accorded human life, any opening
to a new callousness, could have profoundly harmful effects
elsewhere. This argument (like so many others we have seen)
is not a coercive one, but it is one that gives the prudent
person pause as he contemplates the predicament of the
comatose patient, and guards against a too-easy conclusion
that the survival of such an organism is <u>wholly</u> without
value.

<u>Case D:</u> Modern medicine has discovered a great many ways of
prolonging the period of dying. Chemotherapy for certain
sorts of cancer is perhaps the best known, and there are
many surgical procedures which delay onset of death but
cannot restore health. Our fourth case is that of an
incurably ill person whose life may be lengthened by a
particular therapy. There are variations on the case. For
example, there may be a small chance that the therapy may in
fact cure the person. Or the therapy may itself be painful
or disfiguring or enormously expensive or still in an experi-
mental stage. But the "basic" Case D is that of a person
whose life may be prolonged but not saved.

Of all the cases we have considered, it is this one
perhaps which most clearly typifies the ambiguous results
of medical technology, especially of the up-to-date highly
specialized hospital. The aim of such hospitals is to cure.
But failing that, prolonging life can easily seem the next
best goal. If there is a technique that can keep a patient
alive, there will be a natural tendency to try it. But, of
course, trying it may <u>not</u> be in the best interests of the
patient. How are these interests to be determined ?

First, the wishes of the patient himself or herself
must have primary force. It is perfectly proper for someone
to refuse to make use of a life-prolonging manoeuvre. It is
also proper for him to request that every effort be made to
extend his life as long as possible. There can obviously be
a great many reasons that could justify either decision. In
order that the decision may be a good one, the physician has
an obligation to clarify the alternatives as best he can
for the patient. He has to be especially careful to leave
no doubt that the therapy <u>is</u> merely one of prolongation,
and to specify the negative effects that may follow from
its use.

But what if the patient is impaired in judgement, as is
so very often the case with people so gravely ill ? Or what
if he simply leaves it up to the expert to decide, as
patients so often will ? Here the physician has to balance
all the relevant factors: the quality of the life that the

therapy would, if successful, make possible, the possible side-effects of its use, the importance (if it can be assessed) to the patient of extra time, and above all, the patient's temperament. The family will ordinarily be involved in such a decision; it is especially important that this be so nowadays if the malpractice threat is not to become a separate and distorting influence.

There are no clear-cut norms for such a decision; experience and wisdom are needed to assess the various factors and to try to balance them against one another. Case D is of itself relatively uncontroversial: hardly anyone would hold that life ought to be prolonged at all costs. But there are many complicating features that may make decisions extremely difficult to reach. Notable among these is the sheer momentum of medical technology itself, and the tendency on the part of the dying to grasp at straws that in their earlier more rational existence would have been unhesitatingly rejected. Can their wishes in such a case be overruled ? This is one of the most delicate and painful questions a physician can have to face.

Case E: The previous two types of case are to a large extent the product of the rapid advances in medicine of our own century. But what of the case as old as man himself, of someone who is dying in very great pain: is he entitled to shorten his life ? Are others permitted to help him in such an endeavor ? It is understood that he is clear-headed enough to know the significance of what he is doing and that there is no way to alleviate his pain medically. (The "pain" might, by extension, be the bitter indignity of a physical situation that is destroying self-respect). May such a person act to end his life directly, by the use of poison, for example ?

If one were to rely on simple utilitarian norms, the answer would be quick and easy: yes. Even if one takes the happiness of the individual agent as guide, it would still seem that such an action would be sanctioned. Yet in the Western tradition, it would be generally regarded as suicide, and those who co-operated in it would be thought culpable. This is a case which has always troubled Christian moralists, but on which Christian teaching has in the past been un-equivocal. The writers of the Old Testament repeat over and over that the moment of death is in God's hand, not ours. Our life is His giving, and it is His to determine the manner of its taking away. The example of Christ in the New Testament who suffered so terribly in his dying, conveyed very strongly the notion that suffering has a redemptive value, not only for the individual himself but for the community generally. Those who surround the dying person will be ennobled and strengthened by his acceptance of the pain that, in the Providence of God, is his in his last moments. His pain thus takes on a value in the order of salvation, and is not to be regarded simply as an evil.

Needless to say, these ideas encounter strenuous opposition today. For those for whom death marks an absolute termination and not the transition to a fuller life with God, and for whom the notions of Providence and redemption make no sense, a refusal to consider active euthanasia on such grounds would carry no weight. Even outside the Christian context, however, there would not be agreement about the propriety of euthanasia in these circumstances. Resignation in the face of suffering is not characteristic of our activist age; virtue is found in the struggle to overcome the given, rather than its patient acceptance.

Yet it would be hard to deny the wisdom that is born of suffering, and the contribution such wisdom can make to others. In the U.S., death is concealed to such an extent behind the walls of hospitals and funeral parlors that encounter with death is simply not part of the culture. There is an immaturity, a refusal to face the human condition, that observers from other cultures have often noted. Dying people, suffering people, have an important social role to play, one that is now almost entirely denied them in our culture. This is not to say that suffering should not be shortened, when possible. But the fact that it has become such a private and unrecognized affair makes the lot of the dying person far harder to bear.

Case E is simple to state, but on an existential level it is the most harrowing of the five we have described. So much will depend on the patient's earlier experience of suffering, on his attitude towards death, on his readiness for death. We have been discussing the kinds of decision about termination of life that have to be made in the context of medical science. But there is one far more basic sort of decision that faces every dying person; it is the decision to accept death, to close the books peacefully and in confidence. In a symposium about "Death and decision" it is well to recall that <u>this</u> is the crucial decision, and the one hardest to reach.

It will be noted in all five cases outlined above, there are no simple and easily applicable principles that would enable a moralist looking at the type of case to say <u>a priori</u>: this is wrong, or this is right. In each, there are many factors to balance, many intangibles to grope for.

A person's decision about death in the last analysis will be guided by what he, and the others around him, believe the significance of life, and therefore of death, to be. And this is not something easily set down, nor readily universalizable.

Our purpose in this Introduction was to sketch in a summary way some of the dilemmas faced by the dying and by those who care for them. The papers that follow were originally presented at a symposium on "The right to die" at the annual meeting of the American Association for the Advancement of Science in Denver, February 1977. Several of the papers have been extensively reworked for publication. We would like to thank the numerous people who helped in the planning of the original meeting, notably David Solomon, Stanley Hauerwas, Thomas Shaffer, Harold Widdison and Tristram Engelhardt.

It is our hope that this collection of essays may sharpen our thinking on, and heighten our sensitivities to, some of the most difficult and most important areas of moral decision. It is in this border between life and death that the moral quality of a culture perhaps most clearly reveals itself.

1

Definitions of Death: Where to Draw the Lines and Why

H. Tristram Engelhardt, Jr.

Defining death should not be viewed as a mysterious enterprise, despite whatever mysteries we may take to surround death. Such definitions reflect general human purposes and goals. Still, the web of definitions of death is complex and requires analysis. What I will attempt here is a brief sketch of various definitions of death, as well as the presuppositions they involve and the purposes they serve. In that way I hope to show what different definitions of death have at stake, the concerns and commitments in terms of which they function.

In addition, definitions of death are distinguished in terms of the social mediums in which they function--for example, medical, legal, and religious concepts of death do not necessarily denote essentially different concepts, but may instead signal special social circumstances within which definitions of death receive a particular articulation or employment. In many cases both religious and legal definitions of death rely on the accepted medical definitions.[1, 2] In fact, unless religious definitions represent the exegesis of some accepted traditional definition of death,[3] the problem of the definition of death is a mix of philosophical and medical issues. It is a philosophical issue with regard to the conceptual dimension. In order to decide regarding the usefulness of various measures of death, one must decide what one wishes to measure. Only then can one discuss the reliability of various measures of death. It is this latter set of issues, the reliability of operational definitions or measures of death, which is primarily medical. What I will do here is to present some central issues ingredient in choosing among different definitions of death, and then say something about the recent history of the development of the definition of death.

Justifying A Definition of Death

First and foremost, one must ask what purposes a definition of death serves. An answer cannot simply be that a definition functions to let us know when to transfer estates or to remove organs for transplantation--each of these answers begs the point at issue. What is death such that it makes the transfer of estates or removal of organs appropriate? What does it mean to be dead? To begin with, it usually means that one is no longer in the world in the sense that having an estate, keeping one's kidneys, or receiving the last sacraments, is no longer of any direct and immediate significance to the person in question. To be dead is no longer to be around, to be one on whom things in this world can have direct and immediate bearing.

The weight is borne by <u>direct</u> and <u>immediate</u>. Individuals can have concerns about the world as it will exist subsequent to their death. The use of wills, the establishment of trusts for children, and the signing of uniform acts for the donation of organs concern the world after one's death. One can, as well, hope that individuals will keep the promises they make on one's deathbed. At death, when one ceases to experience things in this world, or to act directly upon them, one may continue to act indirectly through various means including legal instruments, but no longer immediately and directly.

Defining death should, in its roots, be a commonsense enterprise. One should be seeking ways of characterizing those states in which almost all of us would see no further sense in being termed 'alive' versus those states in which most of us would see it to be appropriate.[4] We are, though, forced to do philosophical analysis to the extent that the answer to such questions presupposes an understanding of what it means to be a person. In order to decide when we will be dead, we must to some extent reflect on what we are. The examination of the nature of persons in these settings is, thus, an attempt to determine under what circumstances we will cease to be experiencers and agents in this world. The concept of person is here used only by way of exclusion, that is, in order to identify those entities in the world that are neither experiencers nor agents. Depending on what one packs into the concepts experiencer and agent, such a characterization may not specify persons as such: it may include hogs and chickens which both experience and in some limited sense act upon the world.[5] The criteria being advanced may thus not provide unique sufficient conditions for being a person, but provide somewhat non-specific necessary conditions. Moreover,

such conditions may vary in specificity. Both minimal sentience, as well as minimal consciousness, may be necessary conditions for being a person. The second condition,
minimal consciousness (or capacity for consciousness) is the
more specific insofar as consciousness is more peculiar to
persons than sentience.[6]

As a result, there are a variety of answers to the conceptual questions regarding the definition of death, with the
answers varying according to what is taken to count as immediately experiencing and doing in this world. One finds individuals advancing different specific necessary conditions
for the life of a person: (1) mere human biological life,
(2) a minimal degree of sentience, and (3) a minimal level of
consciousness (or capacity for consciousness). These views
come out of a rich history of controversy concerning the
meaning of 'embodiment' and the meaning of 'person'. Two
leitmotifs can be isolated with benefit for the discussion
of the definition of death. The first is the development of
the concept of the cerebral localization of mental functions.
A convenient terminus a quo is the Cartesian portrayal of the
mind acting as a unit upon the brain through the pineal
gland.[7] A convenient terminus ad quem is the view of John
Hughlings Jackson that mental functions can at least be mapped
imprecisely upon the brain.[8] Between these points lie
colorful controversies including disputes between French
neurologists such as Pierre Flourens who in 1845 dedicated
one of his books to the philosophy of Descartes in order to
defend a view of the mind as a unity acting upon the cerebral
hemispheres,[9] and the protagonists of localization of mental
functions such as Franz Josef Gall [10] and Johann Spurzheim.[11]
By the end of the 19th century, a view of the localization of
cerebral functions, as well as a concept of sensory-motor
integration as the physiological equivalent of mental function had become generally accepted by the scientific community.[12] Moreover, distinctions were drawn between higher and
lower brain functions, and these were associated with distinctions between higher and lower mental functions.[13] Some
functions were seen to be more closely associated with the
life of a person than others.

A second and concomitant leitmotif was a move from
identifying the person with a general principle of life, to
identifying the person with a special principle of consciousness. For example, St. Thomas Aquinas had talked of the soul
as being in all its reality, in all the parts of the body--
tota in toto and tota in qualibet parte. At the same time,
it is worth noting St. Thomas distinguished among a nutritive,

a sensitive, and an intellectual soul.[14] The nutritive and
sensitive souls were held to exist in humans prior to the
development of the intellectual soul. Once the intellectual
soul appeared in human ontogeny, however, it was taken to
embrace and include the realities of the nutritive and sensitive souls. As a helpful aside, one should note that
St. Thomas distinguished between early abortions which were
only the taking of biological life, and late abortions which
involved taking the life of a human person.[15] On the basis
of the level of biological organization required for the life
of a person, St. Thomas drew what was tantamount to a distinction between human biological and human personal life--
but at the beginning of the human life cycle. This distinction is helpful because it suggests the usefulness of distinguishing different senses of human life.

Returning to our concern with the end of the human life
cycle, the issue of brain death, one should notice that brain
oriented concepts of death involve an analogous distinction
between mere human biological life and human personal life.
This distinction presupposes the shift in modern thought
regarding the nature of our embodiment, mentioned above, so
that (1) the mind is seen to be associated with particular
parts of the brain, allowing the possibility of distinguishing between the embodiment of higher and lower mental functions, and (2) the person is identified primarily with the
mind, not with a general principle of life, thus further
supporting the singling out of the brain as the special locus
of mental and thus personal activity. These developments
encourage distinguishing personal life from merely biological
life, in the way that the mind became distinguished from a
general principle of life. When such distinctions are
elaborated, one can separate two questions: What is it to
be biologically dead? What is it to be dead as a person?
The first is concerned with the cessation of biological processes, while the second bears the burden of identifying
those activities which make a direct difference for an individual as a sentient or conscious being. Once distinctions
between human biological and human personal life are at hand,
one can argue for whole-brain oriented definitions of death--
or for that matter for neocortical definitions of death.
Moreover, it becomes possible to ask whether one should consider individuals dead in conditions similar to those in
which Karen Quinlan was when her case came to judicial
review.[16]

The presuppositions of whole-brain definitions of death
are, then, (1) that being a person requires some minimal
level of sentience, and (2) that sentience is embodied in the

brain so that destruction of the brain is tantamount to
destruction of the person. In contrast, someone who defended
the whole-body definition of death against the whole-brain
definition would very likely be holding that being a person
is associated with human biological life simpliciter, or that
the person as a receiver of experience and as an initiator
of action was not uniquely embodied in the brain. Further,
those defending neocortical definitions of death[17] (or even
holding individuals in conditions such as Karen Quinlan's to
be dead) would be saying that a necessary and sufficient, or
at least a fairly specific necessary condition for being
alive as a person is some level of consciousness or capacity
for consciousness.

    This latter view of death runs contrary to cliches that
stress that any human life is of absolute value. Instead,
such definitions presuppose that life has no intrinsic value,
only instrumental value, so that when the person living a
life is no longer capable of being conscious, that life
ceases to be of any direct value to him or her--and, he or
she is dead. He or she is no longer living a life, though
biological life may continue. Whatever biological life
remains may or may not have instrumental value for others.
This point can be brought across commonsensically by imagin-
ing one's reaction if a physician were to determine that one
had a serious disease, but that one would not 'die', only
that one's neocortex would be destroyed. One's reaction
would likely be--"Some comfort! Sans neocortex, sans
conscious life, I am no longer around--I am no longer alive."
Or, one need only consider what consolation would be offered
by the assurance that one would 'live' to the age of one
hundred and ten in a condition similar to that reported concerning Karen Quinlan in the New Jersey Superior and Supreme
Court rulings. Again, the reaction is likely to be, and on
good grounds, that such a life would be of no direct significance to the person in question. One would no longer be
an experiencer or an agent in the world. Note, this is not
to say that life for the individual would be too painful,
too deformed, or too boring to live. Rather life would be of
no direct and immediate bearing on that person. In short,
as I have been arguing, that person would be dead. In fact,
as one moves in this direction one comes to define persons
as moral agents or possible members of a moral community--or
at least as humans who can interact within a social context;
that is, as entities for whom the world is recognizable by
them as having bearing upon them, and in which they thus have
responsibilities.[18]

    One can, then, come to determine what one means by the

death of a person through testing what would generally count
as states in which an individual would no longer be a subject
of experience or an agent in this world, where life could not
possibly have any further direct significance to the individual involved. Death of a person would obtain at the point
of sufficient bodily destruction where there is no one alive
to experience anything, with no potential for recovering the
ability to experience or act. The question of potential for
recovery raises concern regarding the trustworthiness of
particular operational concepts of death--not to mention
issues of personal identity. (What does it mean to say that
a person is alive though comatose or even asleep?--probably
that the developed physical basis of that person, his or her
brain, is intact, and that that person can wake up. The
person still has a unique presence in the world which could
allow the person in question to 'regain' consciousness).[19]
After all, we all have an interest in having as few false
positive determinations as possible in tests for death.
Which is to say, even if we were to hold for neocortically
oriented concepts of death on conceptual grounds, we may
still hold to a whole-body oriented concept of death in order
to avoid false positive tests. We have good grounds for
being very careful and conservative in the selection of
operational definitions of death, since being falsely labeled
dead is, quite obviously, of great significance. On the
other hand, we also want to avoid as many false negatives as
possible. We wish to do so, for example, because of the financial and psychological investment which is wasted when one
mistakenly takes dead bodies to be living persons, and on
account of the possible loss of useful organs for transplantation. Still, one will prudently accept some level of
false positives. For example, one false positive in every
million deaths is probably not worth worrying about, especially if many of the individuals so labeled would be severely ill; this makes the mistake often of little significance,
if any, for the persons involved. In any event, one must
assume some risks in order to make decisions in medicine,
and defining death is no exception.

A distinction must, at this point, be made between operational and conceptual definitions of death, a point already
advanced regarding this topic by Leon Kass.[20] Conceptual
definitions of death indicate what we mean by death--for
example, the complete cessation of all biological functions,
or the complete cessation of the life of persons as sentient
beings. Operational definitions indicate how we are to measure what we mean by death--for example, one might use operational definitions based on the cessation of respiration and
heartbeat; or on the absence of (a) response to stimuli, (b)
spontaneous movements including breathing, and (c) brain

mediated reflexes accompanied by a flat EEG. One may have more than one operational definition of death for any one conceptual definition. That is, in most cases it appears sufficient to rely upon cessation of respiration and heart-beat as an operational definition of death, even if one holds that the indices used in whole-brain death are more precise.

One may also have different conceptual definitions of death answering to the characterization of various states of affairs which we may hold to be equivalent to death--for example, conceiving of death as the cessation of human bio-logical life versus holding it to be the cessation of human personal life. Further, there are numerous operational de-finitions of death: whole-body oriented definitions of death, whole-brain oriented definitions of death, and neo-cortically oriented definitions of death (the word 'oriented' is meant to indicate which indices of death signal specific necessary conditions for life).[21] On the other hand, there are several conceptual definitions of death to which the above operational definitions may or may not be related: cellular death, death of the human organism as a biological unit, and death of the human person.

We are thus confronted with the two-fold task of (1) becoming clearer about what we mean by being alive as per-sons, and (2) developing reliable operational definitions of death. Neither of these enterprises should appear as a mysterious or arcane endeavor. They, rather, concern the development of commonsense appreciations of what it means to be in this world, coupled with assessments of the reliability of indicators of the bodily destruction we take to preclude further presence in the world.

A Few Historical Anecdotes

In order to give flesh to these considerations, I will now turn to some historical anecdotes from the development of legal definitions of death. I will address legal defini-tions not in order to illuminate the legal issues themselves, but because the legal history shows in some detail how the considerations I have discussed have been weighed. The tradi-tional attitude in the Anglo-American world with regard to the definition of death was reflected in the fourth edition of Black's Law Dictionary. The definition given in this dictionary incorporated traditional understandings of the criteria for death; it, in turn, was cited in many court cases in order to bolster the whole-body definition of death. The Dictionary defined death as "the cessation of life; the ceas-ing to be; defined by physicians as a total stoppage of the circulation of the blood, and a cessation of the animal and vital functions consequent thereon, such as respiration, pulsation, etc."[22] The force of this traditional definition was that a person should be held to be 'alive' even if the brain were destroyed with the loss of any future possibility of sentient, personal human life. The continuation of biological functions such as respiration, pulsation, and heartbeat are, according to the traditional definition, a sufficient basis for the life of a person.

The whole-body definition of death, which focuses on biological functions, when interpreted as a conceptual definition, produced legal decisions that seem inappropriate if not bizarre. For example, in a Kentucky case in 1952, in which the precise definition of death was of importance for deciding which of two individuals died first, it was held that a decapitated individual outlived another person whose heartbeat had stopped at approximately the time of the first individual's decapitation. Testimony indicated that the first individual was discovered after an auto accident " . . decapitated, her head lying about ten feet from her body, which was actively bleeding "from near her neck and blood was gushing from her body in spurts" . . . .". Physicians in that case informed the court that "a body is not dead so long as there is a heartbeat and that may be evidenced by the gushing of blood in spurts."[23] In short, though the decapitated individual sustained severe cerebral anoxia at the same time, if not earlier, than the individual whose heartbeat had stopped, still she was taken to have lived longer. Similar opinions were reflected in cases in which the court held, for example, as in Arkansas in 1958, that "death occurs precisely when life ceases and does not occur until the heart stops beating and respiration ends."[24] Or, again, the Supreme Court of Kansas in 1967 held that "death is the complete cessation of all vital functions without possibility of resuscitation."[25] The accent on "the complete cessation of all vital functions" raised serious difficulties, for it implied that turning off a ventilator sustaining a brain dead, but otherwise alive body, or removing the heart from such a body, would involve taking the life of a person. As a result, pressure developed to distinguish between personal death and organismic death (i.e., cessation of all vital functions). Further, whole-body oriented definitions of death appeared counter-intuitive—a decapitated body did not easily lend itself to being considered a person. The whole-body definition of death appeared poorly drawn.

The brain-oriented concepts of death with which we have become familiar were developed in order to resolve these problems. The issues were, as the above suggests, wide ranging. They included, to summarize, legal, conceptual, economic and social difficulties: (1) court cases had been decided on grounds which appeared, at least to some individuals, to be misconceived. That is, appeals to whole-body definitions of death in contrast with whole-brain definitions of death appeared to distort reality in that being alive without any sentience did not appear to be the same as being alive as person. (2) There was mounting economic pressure to decide when the continuation of the artificial maintenance of respiration no longer preserved the life of a person, and simply maintained whole-body preparations and (3) the development of the technical ability to transplant organs, in particular non-paired organs, led to pressure to develop definitions of death that would allow the salvage of such organs prior to any ischemic damage. Remedy for these difficulties required finding grounds for declaring individuals dead who were still biologically alive. That is, these problems stimulated attempts to distinguish between human biological and human personal life. Given the characteristics of human life, this required a concept of embodiment which portrayed embodiment as more focused--an account of embodiment which presented persons as primarily associated with their brains, not with their bodies generally. The credibility of this account was illustrated by organ transplantation: there appeared to be no grounds for expecting that the transplantation of any organ except the brain would transplant the person. To recast a phrase from the philosopher Roland Puccetti--where the brain is or is not, the person is or is not.[26]

In 1968 the Ad Hoc Committee of the Harvard Medical School to Examine The Definition of Brain Death proposed a qualified whole-brain oriented definition of death. Rather than wait for whole-body death, they argued for pronouncing an individual dead as soon as such an individual was in a state of irreversible coma.[27] In doing so, the Committee did not advance a definition of brain death in sensu stricto, but rather a definition of irreversible coma. The Committee argued that where there is no possibility of functioning, one should be considered, for all practical purposes, to be dead,[28] and irreversible coma should be taken as a measure of death. There is, though, a danger in such unclarity--namely, that it suggests a confusion of the questions, Whether a person is dead? and Whether it is inappropriate to continue sustaining the life of a person?[29]

In 1969, the Ad Hoc Committee of the American Electroencephalographic Society of EEG Criteria for Determination of Cerebral Death further articulated the Harvard Committee's suggestions, but these were now explicitly understood as indices composing an operational definition of death that distinguished between human biological and human personal life.[30] Unreactive coma, absence of striated muscle activity, an absence of reflexes, and, in particular, brain mediated reflexes, together with electroencephalographic silence (unassociated with such conditions an anesthetic drug levels or pronounced hyporthermia) were accepted as reliable criteria for the death of a person.

With regard to the legal history, it is important to observe that the state of Kansas passed a law[31] in 1968 which, on being revised in 1969[32], became a model for the uniform act for the donation of organs--an act motivated in part, as was the Report of the Harvard Committee, by the burgeoning interest in the 1960's for the transplantation of vital organs. Such interest led in 1970, given the ambiguities of the legal definition of death in Kansas, to Kansas passing the first statutory definition of death, a statute which recognized two operational definition of death: (1) the old whole-body definition, (2) the new brain-oriented definition whose greater precision was useful in cases such as those associated with possible transplantation. In particular, it resolved the tension between the easier availability of organs allowed by the Uniform Act, and the whole-body definition of death. Consider, for example, the wording of the portion of the Kansas Statute concerned with the brain-oriented definition of death:

> A person will be considered medically and legally
> dead if, in the opinion of a physician, based on
> ordinary standards of medical practice, there is the
> absence of spontaneous brain function; and if based
> on ordinary standards of medical practice, during
> reasonable attempts to either maintain or restore
> spontaneous circulatory or respiratory function in
> the absence of aforesaid brain function, it appears
> that further attempts at resuscitation or supportive
> maintenance will not succeed, death will have occurred
> at the time when these conditions first coincide.
> Death is to be pronounced before artificial means
> of supporting respiratory and circulatory function
> are terminated and before any vital organ is removed
> for purposes of transplantation (18).[33]

This definition provided a number of important refinements in the legal understanding of death and the proper treatment of the dying. One of these was the requirement that one pronounce the individual dead and <u>then</u> turn off the respirator--

affirming a distinction between human personal and human
biological life. Thus, turning off a respirator on a brain
dead but otherwise alive body does not count either as euthanasia or letting a person die because there is no person to
let die--the person has already died. Moreover, it does not
confuse criteria for death with criteria for states in which
it is no longer appropriate to extend the life of a patient--
for example, states of irreversible coma which might not meet
all the criteria for death.

Because the Kansas definition offered two ways to
measure death, two operational concepts of death, it was
suggested, by way of ridicule, that there were two ways to
die in Kansas.[34] The correct interpretation in this and
similar statutes is that both a more crude and a more precise
set of determinations are available to suit different circumstances. In sum what is being defined remains the same, i.e.
the death of a person. The brain-oriented concept of death
provides a direct measure of the death of a person, given
the presuppositions regarding embodiment and the meaning of
person which have just been discussed. The whole-body
oriented definition of death provides an indirect means of
measuring the death of the person, since the death of the
body as a whole is a good sign of the death of the brain,
which is tantamount to the death of the person. This is
analogous to the often-encountered case of numerous measures
of varying precision for one condition or state of affairs.
Consider, for example, the difference in precision between
measuring blood pressure by means of a sphygmomanometer
relying upon hearing Korotkoff sounds, versus measurement by
an in-dwelling arterial catheter. In each case what is
measured is the same, though the means of measurement and
their precision varies. One can thus continue to use whole-
body death as the usual operational definition of death even
if one recognizes a superior claim for whole-brain or neocortical oriented definitions of death as conceptual definitions. This is the case for, in most circumstances, there
is no need for the precision of brain-oriented definitions
of death.

The enactment of a statutory definition of death by
Kansas in 1970 was followed by a similar statute in Maryland
in 1972,[35]and then rapidly by numerous other states.[36] In
this regard, it should be noted that some individuals have
pressed for wording statutes in a way that confuses the distinction between human biological and human personal life,
a distinction such statutes presuppose. For example
the New Mexico Statute adopted in 1973 uses the phrase
'human being' rather than 'person,'[37] though the brain dead

but otherwise alive individual remains in many respects a
human being--such an individual, for example, could continue
to produce sperm so as to be cross-fertile with members of
our species, etc. That is, it remains an instance of human
biological life.

With the establishment of the whole-brain concept of
death, some have argued that this measure itself is too crude
and imprecise. They have contended that the operational
definition of the death of a person should be based upon
neocortical, not total brain death, because the neocortex is
the seat of consciousness and other essential attributes of
being a person.[38,39] Reliable ways have thus been sought
for declaring a person dead, given an isoelectric spontaneous electroencephalogram and unremitting coma, even with the
presence of spontaneous respiration, tendon reflexes, and
extensor plantar reflexes. Again, what is being argued is
that reasonable and prudent persons would not consider that
they had been offered greater life span with the prospect of
the survival of their body, given the destruction of their
neocortex.

The conceptual distinction between human personal life
and human biological life thus invites ever more precise
operational definitions of death as long as these are consistent with the well founded concern to avoid false positive
determinations of death. Which is to say, given the success
of these conceptual distinctions, the only appropriate arguments against neocortical definitions of death would be in
terms of the lack of reliability of the operational indices
that would be required for their determination.

Some Concluding Reflections

In developing concepts of death, I take it that we have
at least four goals in mind: (1) to develop sufficiently
clear conceptual definitions of death so that we can understand when it no longer makes sense to speak of ourselves as
being in this world, (2) to develop effective operational
definitions that will allow us to identify the physical
states that the conceptual definitions presuppose so that we
will not be subjected to the parody of being kept "alive"
after the cessation of our lives as persons, (3) to distinguish between human personal life and human biological life
so that scarce resources are not invested in supporting
human biological life under the misconception that it is
still human personal life (false negative determinations of
health) as well as to allow the organs of brain dead but
biologically alive individuals to be made available to help

persons who are alive, and (4) to insure accuracy in operational definitions of death so that they do not produce a sufficiently high number of false positives to justify concern with regard to our own safety.

These issues are basic to understanding what it would mean, using Ramsey's cliche,[40] to treat patients as persons. On the one hand, we wish to accord special dignity and respect to the rights of persons. On the other hand, we do not want to confuse persons with things, including merely biologically alive things. Definitions of death serve this social role so that one can distinguish between stealing an organ from a living person and harvesting an organ from a dead person. Moreover, as I stressed above, one must keep clearly in mind the distinction between defining death and developing criteria to identify the inappropriateness of further support of life.

We are left then with the problem of becoming clearer about when it makes sense to say a person is dead and determining reliable criteria to identify the physical destruction associated with such a state. The first is a conceptual problem. The second is, in part, a question of technology, of developing more precise operational definitions (i.e., ones focused not just on the physical basis of sentience, but on that of consciousness) requiring more exquisite diagnostic maneuvers. It is also a question of prudence, of how many false positives one will tolerate in order to avoid false negatives. Insofar as it becomes clear that being alive as a person is not the same as being alive as, say, Karen Quinlan is alive, we will find ourselves pressed further in our pursuit of more precise definitions of both persons and the nature of death. These are enterprises of singular intellectual and practical interest.

Footnotes

1. The tenor of Pope Pius XII's opinion concerning the
    definition of death, though ambiguous, appears to show
    a great reliance on medical opinion. See Pope Pius XII,
    "The Prolongation of Life," in The Pope Speaks 4 (1958),
    393-98.

2. Many legal opinions, including those for whole-body
    death, appear to be based on general medical opinion,
    for example: W. Curran and E. Shapiro, Law, Medicine
    and Forensic Science (Boston: Little, Brown and Co.,
    1970), pp. 940-42.

3. See, for example, Immanuel Jakobovits, Jewish Medical
    Ethics (New York: Block Pub. Co., 1959) p. 277; also
    Tzitz Eliezer, 9:46 and 10:25:4, and Babylonian Talmud,
    Yoma 85a, Soncino Edition.

4. Decisions in a pluralist society properly reflect what
    the majority of individuals in that society agree to be
    the case or agree to let experts determine is the case,
    without appeal to transcendent realities (e.g., revealed
    religion). This point, though, can also be made con-
    ceptually in terms of the hypothetical viewpoint of a
    reasonable and prudent person. A society may, however,
    not agree with what reasonable and prudent persons
    would hold to be the case; that is, a society may not
    be reasonable and prudent. Insofar as one has concep-
    tual interests in mind, the latter criteria will suffice.
    Insofar as one has the political acceptability of de-
    finitions of death in mind, the former criteria will
    need to be invoked.

5. The issue of what counts as being an experiencer and an
    agent in the world is core to understanding the meaning
    of embodiment. H. Tristram Engelhardt, Jr., Mind-Body:
    A Categorical Relation (The Hague, Netherlands:
    Martinus Nijhoff, 1973).

6. The ambiguities in our use of 'person' have marked
    consequences for our treatment of animals and humans.
    If one uses 'person' in a strict sense so as to denote
    'moral person' (i.e. those individuals whom one could
    not use as means merely without rejecting the moral
    order), it would follow that some humans are not persons
    (e.g., brain dead but otherwise alive humans and human
    fetuses) and that perhaps some persons are not humans
    (e.g., extraterrestrial self-conscious life, gods, and

angels). In fact, 'person' in a strict sense may
include some higher primates or dolphins.
The point is that insofar as 'person' functions to sort
out those entities to which one owes unqualified
respect, it is not clear that one includes under that
rubric small infants or the very senile. Consider, for
example, Immanuel Kant's definition of person: "Rational beings are designated as persons." (Immanuel Kant,
Foundations of the Metaphysics of Morals, trans. by
L. W. Beck [New York: Bobbs-Merrill, 1969], p. 53;
Akademie Textausgabe, Band IV, 428.) Similarly, Rawls
notes that only those entities that can construe their
conduct by reference to the original position can count
as persons. "Moral persons are distinguished by two
features: first they are capable of having (and are
assumed to have) a conception of their good (as expressed
by a rational plan of life); and second they are
capable of having (and are assumed to acquire) a sense
of justice, a normally effective desire to apply and
to act upon the principles of justice, at least to a
certain minimum degree. We use the characterization of
the persons in the original position to single out the
kind of beings to whom the principles chosen apply."
(John Rawls, A Theory of Justice [Cambridge, Mass.:
Belknap Press, 1971], p. 505). Rawls attempts to blunt
the consequences of this definition of person by appeal-
ing to the capacity or potentiality to engage in such
activity. But he does not provide an account of such
capacity or potentiality nor is it clear that such an
account could be given (H. Tristram Engelhardt, Jr.,
"The Ontology of Abortion," Ethics 84 [April 1974],
217-34.)
It is probably the case that we have more than one
concept of person (i.e., in addition to the strict concept of person--as an individual self-conscious, rational,
moral agent, who is a bearer of rights and duties),
in particular, a social sense of person. The latter
sense would identify instances of human life to which
one imputes the rights but not the duties of persons in
order to support and nurture kindness and sympathy
towards the young, the helpless and the old. Such usages
of 'person' would be justified in terms of the general
utility of the consequences of such practices. See
H. Tristram Engelhardt, Jr., "On the Bounds of Freedom:
From the Treatment of Fetuses to Euthanasia,"
Connecticut Medicine 40 [January, 1976], 51-54, 57.
Given a social concept of person by which one would
impute the rights of persons to any human capable of some
minimum level of interaction with normal adult humans

thus sustaining a human social role, for example
of 'child' or 'grandfather', one would wish to use similar criteria for the death of children and the senile
as for adults. That is, if one used neocortical defini-
itions of death one would hold both newborn infants and
normal adults to be alive given neocortical function,
even though the significance of that function would be
quite different in the case of infants (i.e., who would
not be rational enough to be moral agents) than in the
case of adults (where neocortical function can be an
index of the mental abilities requisite for being a
moral agent). Thus, one could use the same criteria
for the rather severely mentally retarded as for normal
adult humans, pace Joseph Fletcher. See, for example,
Joseph Fletcher, "Indicators of Humanhood: A Tentative
Profile of Man," The Hastings Center Report 2 [November,
1972], 1-4 and "Four Indicators of Humanhood--The
Inquiry Matures," The Hastings Center Report 4
[December, 1974], 4-7. Also, H. Tristram Engelhardt,Jr.,
"Some persons are humans, some humans are persons, and
the world is what we persons make of it," in Philosophical Medical Ethics: Its Nature and Significance, edited
by Stuart F. Spicker and H. Tristram Engelhardt, Jr.
(Dordrecht, Holland: D. Reidel Pub. Co., 1977), pp.
183-194.

7. René Descartes, Treatise of Man, trans. by T.S. Hall
    (Cambridge, Mass.: Harvard University Press, 1972), pp.
    86,95,103.

8. H. Tristram Engelhardt, Jr., "John Hughlings Jackson and
    the Mind-Body Relation," Bulletin of the History of Med-
    icine 49 (Summer, 1975), 137-151.

9. M.J.P. Flourens, Examen de la Phrenologie, 2nd ed.
    (Paris: Paulin, 1845).

10. Francois Joseph Gall, On the Functions of the Brain and
    of Each of Its Parts: with Observations on the Possi-
    bilities of Determining the Instincts, Propensities, and
    Talents, or the Moral and Intellectual Dispositions of
    Men and Animals, by the Configuration of the Brain and
    Head, trans. by Winslow Lewis (Boston: Marsh, Capen and
    Lyon, 1835).

11. J. G. Spurzheim, Phrenology or the Doctrine of the
    Mental Phenomena (Boston: Marsh, Capen and Lyon, 1833),
    in two volumes.

12. Robert M. Young, Mind, Brain and Adaptation in the

Nineteenth Century (Oxford: Clarendon Press, 1970).

13. John Hughlings Jackson, "Remarks on Evolution and Dis-
    solution of the Nervous System," in Selected Writings
    of John Hughlings Jackson (London: Staples Press,
    1958), pp. 76-91.

14. St. Thomas Aquinas, Summa Theologica I, Q118, article 2,
    reply to objection 2.

15. St. Thomas Aquinas, Opera Omnia XXVI, In Aristoteles
    Stagiritae, Politicorum seu de Rebus Civilibus (Paris,
    1875) Vives, Book VII, Lectio XII, p. 484.

16. In the matter of Karen Quinlan, No. C-201-75 (New
    Jersey Superior Court, Nov. 10, 1975) :18-19 and In the
    matter of Karen Quinlan, 355 A. 2d 647,660 (New Jersey
    Supreme Court, March 31, 1976).

17. See J. Fletcher, "New definitions of death," Prism 2
    (January, 1974), 13; Adams Brierley, J. B. Brierley,
    J. H. Adams, D. I. Graham, and T. A. Simpson, "Neocorti-
    cal death after cardiac arrest," Lancet 2 (September,
    1971), 560 and A. Rot and H.A.H. van Till, "Letter,"
    Lancet 2 (November, 1971), 1099.

18. In the case of humans which had been persons strictly,
    criteria that would declare non-conscious humans dead
    would be directly focused upon defining the death of
    moral persons in the strict sense. In the case of
    infants recognized as persons in the social sense (e.g.,
    as instances of human life to whom rights are imputed
    because of the general utility of such practices), one
    would be accepting the integrity of brain tissue with
    the possibility to support consciousness as the crite-
    rion for the life of a 'person'. Thus one could on
    those grounds consistently call an infant a living
    person although function of brain tissue in the case of
    infants would not signal the presence of a moral person
    in the strict sense. Moreover, since the line drawn
    socially between persons and non-persons is drawn in
    terms of general consideration of utility, this line
    could be drawn at birth and thus in no way preclude
    abortions by investing fetuses with the status of
    persons.

19. Being a person is thus not like being a thing as a rock
    is a thing. Rocks are always simply there as rocks,
    while persons only at times do those things which single
    them out as persons. They sleep, and thus cease to act

as moral agents. Yet as long as a particular person
has come into existence and can continue to unite
further memories under the same 'I think', one would
have grounds for saying that that person continues
through time even if the segments of that person's life
are broken by sleep or coma. But, not only does physical
continuity of a brain appear, at least in part, to be a
necessary condition for personal identity, it appears
as well in usual circumstances to be a sufficient condition. That is, once a person has come into existence,
and in a sense has taken possession of a particular
brain (i.e., in that that brain is the physical presence of that individual), there is a sense to speaking
of that person being there even while asleep or in a
coma.
In order not to obscure both conceptual and practical
issues (e.g., abortion) one would have to distinguish
between the potentiality to become a person and the
capacity of a person to regain consciousness (i.e., in
the latter case there would have already been a person
concerning whom it would make sense to say that his or
her brain was alive and that he or she could awaken).
Here also one should approach the analysis of the meaning of concepts in a commonsensical fashion. We have
an idea of what it would mean to say that Joe is still
alive though asleep or in a coma as long as Joe's brain
is still intact, in a way in which it would not make
sense to talk of what Joe did, for example, as a zygote
(concerning zygotes we do not know who they will turn
out to be).

20. L. R. Kass, "Death as an event: A commentary on Robert
     Morison," Science 173 (August, 1971), 698.

21. Robert M. Veatch, "Choosing Not to Prolong Dying,"
     Medical Dimensions 40 (December, 1972), 8-10.

22. Black's Law Dictionary, 4th ed. rev. (St. Paul, Minn.:
     West Pub. Co., 1968).

23. Grey et al. v. Sawyer et al., Grey et al., v., Clay et
     al., 247 S.W. 2d 496, 497 (Ky.App. 1952).

24. Smith v. Smith, 229 Ark. 576, 317 S.W. 2d 275 (1958).

25. United Trust Company v. Pyke, 199 Kan. 1, 427 P. 2d. 67,
     71 (1967).

26. R. Puccetti, "Brain transplantation and person iden-
     tity," Analysis 29 (January, 1969), 65

27. Ad Hoc Committee of the Harvard Medical School to
     Examine the Definition of Brain Death, "A Definition of
     Irreversible Coma," Journal of the American Medical
     Association 205 (August, 1968), 337.

28. Ibid, p. 337

29. Robert M. Veatch, "Choosing Not to Prolong Dying,"
     Medical Dimensions 40 (December, 1972), 8-10, 40.

30. The Ad Hoc Committee of the American Electroencephalo-
     graphic Society on EEG Criteria for Determination of
     Cerebral Death, "Cerebral Death and the Encephalogram,"
     Journal of the American Medical Association 209
     (September, 1969), 1505.

31. (1968) Kansas Session Laws, ch. 63, ᙭1-8.

32. (1969) Kansas Session Laws, ch. 301, ᙭10; Kansas Stat-
     utes Ann. 65-3210 (1969) "Uniform Anatomical Gift Act"
     was approved by the Commissioners on Uniform State Laws
     on July 30, 1968. Curran and Shapiro, n.2 p.931. For
     a discussion of the development of definitions of death
     under the influence of interests such as transplantation
     see Alexander M. Capron and Leon R. Kass,"A Statutory
     Definition of the Standards for Determining Death: An
     Appraisal and a Proposal," University of Pennsylvania
     Law Review 121 (November, 1972), 87-118.

33. Law of Mar. 17, 1970, ch. 378, [1970], Kan. Laws 994
     (codified at Kan. Stat. Ann. ᙭77-202 (Supp. 1971).

34. J. M. Kennedy, "The Kansas Statute of Death - an
     Appraisal," New England Journal of Medicine 285
     (October, 1971), 946-50.

35. Law of May 26, 1972, ch. 693 [1972] Maryland House Bill
     No. 104 (codified at Maryland Ann. Code, Art. 43,
     ᙭54F). (Supp. 1972).

36. Alaska Sess. Laws Ann., ch. 8, ᙭1 [1974] Code of Civil
     Procedure ᙭09.65.120 (1975); Law of September 27, 1974,
     Ch. 1524 [1974] California Assembly Bill No. 3560 (codi-
     fied at California Health and Safety Code, Div. 7, pt.
     1, ch. 3.7) (1974); Law of April 28, 1975, ch. 88-17
     [1975] Georgia Senate Bill No. 106, General Assembly
     Act 745 (codified at Georgia Code 88-1715. 1-2)(1975);
     Law of September 11, 1975, ch. 3, ᙭2 ᙭᙭542 [1975]
     Illinois House Bill No. 1369, Public Act 79-952

(codified as amendment to Uniform Anatomical Gift
Act of September 11, 1969, ¥2) (1975); Regular
Session Law 1975, ch. 2, code tit. 1, bk. 1, tit. 9
[1975] Louisiana Senate Bill No. 533 (new ch. No. 2
codified at Louisiana Revised Statutes of 1950, code
tit. 1, bk. 1, tit. 9, ¥111-3) (1975); Law of July 14,
1975, ¥326.1-.21 [1970] Michigan House Bill No. 4653,
Public Act 158 (new ¥326.1-.21 of the Compiled Laws of
1970) (1975); Law of March 26, 1973, ch. 168 [1973] New
Mexico House Bill No. 260 (codified as new ¥1-2-2.2,
New Mexico Stat. Ann. of 1953) (1973); Law of July 2,
1975, ch. 565 [1975] Oregon House Bill No. 2648 (codified at Oregon Rev. Stat. ch. 565, ¥1) (1975); Law of
March 29, 1976, ch. 780 [1976] Tennessee House Bill No.
1919 (codified at Tennessee Public Laws, ch. 780,
¥1-2) (1976); Law of March 13, 1973, ch. 252 [1973]
Virginia General Assembly Act 1727 (codified to amend
the code of Virginia by adding ¥32-364.3:1) (1973).

37. Law of March 26, 1973, ch. 168 [1973] New Mexico House
     Bill No. 260 (codified as new ¥1-2-2.2, New Mexico
     Stat. Ann. of 1953) (1973).

38. Editorial, Lancet 2 (September, 1971), 590.

39. A report by the Task Force on Death and Dying of the
     Institute of Society, Ethics and the Life
     "Refinements in Criteria for the Determination of
     Death: An Appraisal," Journal of the American Medical
     Association 221 (July, 1972), 51.

40. Paul Ramsey, The Patient as Person (New Haven: Yale
     University Press, 1970).

2

What Is the Function
of Medicine?[1]

Eric J. Cassell

Thought about the care of dying patients has changed
over the past several decades. The questions raised initially concerned physicians' obligations towards the dying.
As the technical power of medical practice increased,
thought was given as to whether "ordinary" or "extraordinary"
means must be used to keep the terminally ill alive. In
more recent times, the emphasis has shifted from the obligations of physicians, to the patient as a possessor of rights.
A glance at bibliographies of bioethics will show the same
increasing preoccupation with the rights of the sick in all
areas of medical care. Whether one sees the topic of the
dying patient from the point of view of physicians'
obligations or patients' rights, it is clearly concerned
with the doctor-patient relationship. I am going to examine
the issue of the patient's right to be allowed to die to
see what it can tell us about the doctor-patient relationship and equally what it can reveal about the intimately
related question - what is the function of medicine?

It is. reasonable to start by seeing what universe of
patients we are talking about. It seems to me that we are
talking about three classes of patients. First are those
patients whose disease is completely curable but if untreat-
ed will probably be fatal. The serious infectious diseases
such as the bacterial meningitides or septicemias come to
mind as examples. But also included would be surgical emer-
gencies such as hemorrhage, shock, head injuries or perfor-
ated ulcers.

A second group of patients are those whose disease is
not curable but who will, with continued treatment, live in
functional health for a variable but meaningful time. In
this class are patients with heart failure, certain malig-
nancies such as Hodgkins' disease, patients with end-stage
renal disease who require regular dialysis with the artifi-

cial kidney, and persons with certain chronic anemias who
need repeated transfusions. This class of patients is ex-
panding as more cancers become responsive to chemotherapy
and other diseases are controlled by newer therapy. The
key characteristics of these patients is not simply that
they live longer but that they require continuing treatment
to remain alive.

The final group are the terminally ill. Their disease
is not curable, and treatment offers nothing beyond the prolongation of their dying.

Although it is the contributions of technology and physicians to the sufferings of this latter group, paradoxi-
cally, that initially raised the issues I am examining, the
question of the patient's right to be allowed to die was
gradually extended to the former two groups in both theory
and practice.

An example from each of the first two groups should
help unpack the issues.

A thirty-eight year old man who had a mild upper res-
piratory infection suddenly developed severe headache, stiff
neck, and a high fever. He went to a local emergency room
for help. Brief examination confirmed the physician's suspicion that the man had meningitis. Based on the story of
the illness and the age of the patient, the most likely
diagnosis was pneumococcal meningitis. This kind of bacterial meningitis is almost uniformly fatal if not treated,
and if simple antibiotic treatment is delayed, although cure
will result, permanent neurological damage is likely. The
doctor told the patient the problem and how important urgent
treatment was to save his life and forestall brain damage.
The patient refused consent for treatment saying that he
wanted to be allowed to die.

Does such a patient have a right to be allowed to die?
On the face of it the answer must be yes. That is because
the patient cannot be legally treated without his consent.
But I would guess that it would be a rare hospital where
such a patient would not be treated against his will. The
physicians would ask for a psychiatric consultation to de-
clare the patient incompetent and then start therapy. Since
penicillin works equally well against the bacteria whether
the patient wants to die or not, he would recover.

Why is my expectation (and sincere hope) that such a
patient would be treated despite his declared wish to be
allowed to die? When a patient enters the hospital (or doc-

tor's office) for help, he enters into a relationship with
the treating physicians -- and by extension the hospital itself. While the nature of that relationship is still obscure, we know that when the physician enters the relationship he acquires a responsibility for the patient that <u>can-
not</u> be morally relieved merely by the patient's refusal to
consent for treatment. But more simply, the physician could
not stand aside and allow the patient to die from a disease
otherwise easily treated without feeling that he, the doctor,
was responsible for the death. Much is said of the patient's rights in the doctor-patient relationship, but the
patient also has obligations. In giving himself into the
responsibility of another, he is obligated not to injure
the other morally or legally by making it impossible for the
physician to act on the responsibility. In coming into the
emergency room for help (he could have <u>not come</u> at all) he
caused the physician and the hospital to become responsible
for him without beforehand limiting the nature and degree
of their responsibility. Although not meaningful in this
case, such antecedent limits might allow the physician to
refuse to enter the relationship.

    In the situation I have described, by refusing treat-
ment, the patient is effectively committing suicide. As opposed to going out a high window, here he is enlisting the
aid of others in his suicide. On the other hand, if he is
not committing suicide, his motives are not clear. Therefore, if he resists treatment, the doctors might reasonably
believe that the patient does not know what he is doing.
The element of time appears to play a part. But time for
what? A different but similar situation may make clear what
function time serves and what is lacking in this case of the
man with meningitis.

    A Jehovah's Witness, injured in an accident, comes to
the hospital bleeding profusely. Blood transfusions are
necessary to save the patient's life before surgery can be
done to stop the bleeding. The Jehovah's Witness refuses
transfusions. While there will probably be much agonizing
over the decision, or even recourse to the courts, the patient's right to refuse treatment (even though death will
follow) may be -- indeed has been, acknowledged. The situations are similar. The condition is curable, but without
treatment death results. What is very different is that
the patient's motive is well known to us and has been expressed by a durable agent, his church, over time. Further,
the patient's decision is consistent with a set of beliefs
well known to us, whatever we may think about them.

    In addition to highlighting the element of time in

allowing the reason for the decision to be expressed over
time, time to be durable and time to be known to us, the
case makes another important point. The Jehovah's Witness
did not ask to be allowed to die, he asked to be permitted
to refuse treatment. That the decision may result in his
death is not relevant. It is not death that is chosen, it
is treatment (and its effects - religious in this instance)
that is being refused. We do not say that the soldier on
a hazardous mission chose death, we say that he was coura-
gous. On reflection, I think that you will see that most,
if not all, instances chosen to highlight the discussion of
patients' rights to die in medical care are instances of
the right to refuse the consequences of treatment of which
death may be only one, and the least important at that.

     From the first group of patients, those whose disease
is curable but who will die without treatment, I must conclude from my experience of how medicine is practiced in
the United States that the patient's right to be allowed to
die will not be honored and that the thing truly being
requested is the right to refuse treatment. Further, at
least one reason the request will not be granted is that
insufficient time is present to assess the patient's
motives if they are not otherwise clear.

     I believe the issues will be clarified by considering
the second class of patients, those whose disease is not
curable but for whom continued treatment will provide
functional life over a long period. As I noted earlier,
this class of patients is daily enlarged by medical advances,
as chronic diseases from cancer to emphysema are more suc-
cessfully treated. Instead of the man with bacterial meningitis, let us pose the case of a patient with sickle cell
anemia requiring repeated transfusions, or a patient with
chronic renal failure who needs dialysis with an artificial
kidney several times weekly. If such a patient were to refuse treatment could the same course be followed as with
the man in the emergency room? It seems unlikely. It has
been the case that a patient who refused further artificial
kidney dialysis was declared incompetent on the basis of
the fact that his refusal constituted suicide. But what
happened then? Did the doctors in that kidney unit tie
him down on the dialysis couch time after time and week after week? If it was a patient with anemia who required continued transfusions, would the doctors force the transfusions on the patient? Again and again and again? That seems
counter-intuitive. But if it is not reasonable, why not?

     These patients, also, presented themselves for treat-
ment and entered into a relationship with a physician and

hospital. That relationship involved the doctor's responsibility and the patient's obligation. However, there are several crucial differences between situations like this and those represented by the man with meningitis. In this instance when the patient refuses treatment and asks to be allowed to die, can we claim that he does not know what he is doing? Obviously not. Patients with chronic diseases requiring long-term therapy are usually very knowledgeable. They have had plenty of time to learn about the disease, its treatment, and the consequences of both disease and treatment. Such patients learn from books, from physicians and nurses, and perhaps most importantly from other patients. Not only is the information available, but, the patient has time to test his beliefs against time and the arguments of others. Certainly at the point of refusing further therapy the patient will be exposed to considerable argument and discussion that can test his reasons and reasoning. The process is two-sided. As the patient has had time to acquire knowledge and test his beliefs, his doctors have had time to know the patient. During the weeks, months, or years that they have been treating him, the staff has an opportunity to know whether the patient's refusal of treatment and desire to die is consonant with all the other things they know of him.

When the man with meningitis refuses treatment and asks to be allowed to die, it does not appear to me to be a truly autonomous act. However, when dialysand refuses further dialysis, his action appears to me to be much more the exercise of his autonomy. To clarify my reasoning it is necessary to look more closely at the concept of autonomy as it applies to medical care. As these last decades have seen the emphasis shift, in the critical and theoretical examination of medicine, from the doctor's obligations to the patient's rights, there has been increasing discussion of the importance of the patient's autonomy. Autonomy appears to be the basis for the demand for informed consent. Patients' autonomy is also, it seems to me, the basis of the move to demystify medicine and make the patient a partner in his or her care. As a society we have come to place increasing value on autonomy. Indeed we often mark ourselves in part by our autonomy. But what is autonomy?

Gerald Dworkin argues (2) that autonomy requires both authenticity and independence. Authenticity is the true selfness of a person. The degree to which their beliefs, ideas or actions are truly their ideas, beliefs or actions despite whatever source they may have had. Someone is authentic to the degree that they are uniquely themselves.

Independence, it appears to me, is above all freedom of
choice. Freedom of choice requires three things: first,
knowledge about the area where choice is to be made. One
cannot be considered to be making a free choice if he does
not know what the choices are. Knowledge alone is not sufficient. To have freedom of choice one must also be able
to reason, to think clearly, otherwise the knowledge is of
little use. Finally, one must have the ability to act on
one's choice, otherwise freedom of choice is meaningless.

When philosophers and lawyers (and many others) talk
about rights they often speak as though the body does not
exist. When they discuss the rights of patients they act
as if a sick person is simply a well person with an illness
appended. Like putting on a knapsack, the illness is added
but nothing else changes. That is simply a wrong view of
the sick. The sick are different than the well (3) to a
degree dependent on the person, the disease, and the circumstances in which they are sick and/or are treated.

Let us see what autonomy means to a sick person, or
conversely what does illness do to autonomy. Let me start
with authenticity. Is an ugly Paul Newman authentic? Am
I my authentic self as I writhe in pain? Am I my authentic
self when I am foul-smelling from vomitus or feces, lying
in the mess of my illness? It is common to hear patients
say that they do not want visitors "to see me like this."
In the first days after a mastectomy, it seems reasonable
when the patient questions her authenticity -- after all,
body-image helps make up our authentic self. And, finally,
is that my authentic father lying there, hooked up to tubes
and wires, weak and powerless? It is clear that illness
can impair authenticity.

But if illness has an effect on authenticity, what does
it do to independence? If freedom of choice requires knowledge, then the sick do not have the same freedom of choice
as the well. Knowledge, for the sick person, is incomplete
and (for the very sick) never can be complete even if the
patient is a physician. For even the best understood disease there are large gaps in understanding. Causes may be
obscure and outcomes vary in probability. But the sick person cannot deal in percentages when what is wanted is certainty. For the doctor caring for the patient, these gaps
are of less importance and uncertainty is his constant
companion. Besides, as Jerimiah Berondess has pointed out,
it is vastly easier for a physician to know what to do than
to know what is the matter.

Not only is knowledge lacking for the sick person but

reason is also impaired. In the simplest terms, it is difficult to be clear headed in pain or suffering. I have
said previously that the very sick may have impairment in
the ability to reason abstractly even when their mental
function is seemingly intact (4). Thus not only is knowledge incomplete for the ill, but the capacity to operate
on the knowledge is disturbed. The final element necessary
for meaningful free choice is the ability to act. Illness
so obviously interferes with the ability to act as to require almost no comment. It should be pointed out, however,
that a patient does not have to be bedridden to be unable
to act, the fear of action born of uncertainty may be just
as disabling.

It is reasonable to conclude that illness interferes
with autonomy to a degree dependent on the nature and severity of the illness, the person involved, and the setting.
The sick person is deprived of wholeness by the loss of
complete independence and by the loss of complete authenticity. What helps restore wholeness? It should first be
pointed out that autonomy is a relational term. Autonomy
is exercised in relation to others; it is encouraged or
defeated by the action of others as well as by the actor.
For this reason wholeness can be restored to the sick (in
the terms of autonomy) in part by family and friends. However, there are limits to the capacity of family or friends
in returning autonomy to the sick, particularly in acute
illness. This is true of both terms of autonomy, authenticity and independence. This is because the well, even
the most loving well, are forced to turn aside from the
ugliness, foulness, pain and suffering of sickness. Merely
the smell of illness and its mess is difficult to surmount
for most people. They are unable to see the sick person in
the bed completely apart from the illness and when sickness
itself does not turn them aside, the setting will. Visitors
in intensive care areas commonly cannot decide where to
look and often end up staring more at the monitors and the
equipment than at the patient. That person on the bed is
simply not the authentic loved one, friend, or relative.
These things are especially true during acute illness although when sickness lasts longer the family may success-
fully overcome their distaste. But further the family is
also injured by damaged authenticity of the beloved sick
person. As the sick person is not whole, neither are they.
Similarly family and friends cannot usually restore independence to the sick person. They, too, do not have the
knowledge of the illness and although they can supply the
ability to reason, their thinking is also clouded by emotion -- by fear, concern, and doubt. Finally, while the
family and friends can (and usually do) provide some surro-

gate ability to act for the sick person, they, like he, cannot act against the most important thief of autonomy, the illness.

There is one relationship from which wholeness can be returned to the patient and that is the relationship with the doctor. The doctor-patient relationship can be the source from which both authenticity and independence can be returned to the patient. The degree of restoration will depend on both patient and doctor and is subject to the limits imposed by the disease. I am also well aware that by his actions or lack of them, the physician can further destroy rather than repair the patient's autonomy. But here I am not speaking of what harm can be done but what good can be done. In the same manner, when I speak of the use of a good and potent drug, I would not focus on its misuse even though it may often be misused, nor concentrate primarily on its side effects, but speak rather of how it can and should be employed.

The physician, in his relationship with the patient, can help restore authenticity. The mess of illness does not repel him and through training he is protected from defensiveness at the pain of others. For these reasons, he can see the person amidst and within the illness. He can see a parent where there is a father or a craftsman, attorney or mother, all aside from the sickness surrounding them. If he has known the patient for a long time he knows the person has a history or he can construct that history from conversation. He has the ability to talk of the future if he chooses (as in all of this) to use that ability. He helps restore authenticity by teaching the sick person how to reassert himself above his disability, by teaching how to be whole when the body is not whole.

The physician can also help return independence to the patient. He has the knowledge of the disease and the circumstances that the patient and family lack and he can search out the knowledge of the person that is necessary to make his medical knowledge meaningful to the patient. He can supply the ability to reason and help bridge the gaps in the patient's ability to reason. Finally, he can provide surrogate ability to act, against the illness if nowhere else. In so doing, the patient can be shown how to act in his own behalf and by that means reach a measure of control over his circumstances.

I must stop now and ask the central question raised by the issue of the patient's right to be allowed to die or

right to refuse the consequences of treatment. Is the function of medicine to preserve biological life or is the function of medicine to preserve the person as he defines
himself?

I believe that the function of medicine is to preserve
autonomy and that preservation of life is neither primary
nor secondary but rather subservient to the primary goal.
This issue is confused by several factors. First, it is
obvious that the best way to preserve autonomy is to cure
the patient of the disease that impairs autonomy and return
him to his normal life. In normal life, doctors and medical
care are irrelevant. The second thing that confuses the
issue is that the threats to life and well-being, and therefore autonomy, have been organized into a system of knowledge and a mode of thought called medical science which
centers around concepts of disease. Doctors are trained to
concentrate on disease and the system of thought, often
forgetting the origins of the system in the human condition.
That body of medical science and the derivative technology
has acquired an existence now independent of its original
function - understanding the sicknesses which rob persons
of their independence and authenticity. The issue is further confused because in the last few centuries of the
history of medicine, the underlying focus of medicine has
been the preservation of the body and biological life. But
until the last two generations it did not matter what the
philosophy was, the tools of medical practice were so poor
that medical care (although perhaps not surgery) had to
function through the agency of the patient. The patient
did or did not follow the regimen or work with the physician. The major tool of medicine was the doctor-patient
relationship itself. Where that is the case, to preserve
the relationship, to keep it functioning,requires the active
participation of the patient. Where the patient's function
is necessary, so is some measure of his autonomy represented.
And it does not matter here whether the patient's autonomy
was expressed primarily by the patient or, primarily by the
physician, so long as the actions and outcome were authentic
to the patient, or at least perceived by the patient as
authentic to himself. That may be difficult to conceive in
this era of "I can do it myself" but is, I believe, supportable from the perspective of previous eras. But, in this
time of technological effectiveness, life at all costs seems
to be a slogan and becomes a reality in the face of which
autonomy is easily destroyed. This last thirty or forty
years of medical history should not be allowed to eclipse
the goals of the previous two thousand years. For me, and
I believe, for most of the history of medicine, the function
of medicine is the preservation of autonomy.

Let us return to the cases. The patient with pneumococcal meningitis is treated against his will (correctly,
I think) because the physicians have not had time to know
whether his desire to avoid treatment is authentic while
they do know it to be suicidal. Further, the only consequences of treatment that can be perceived are a return
to health. It appears reasonable to me that where doubt
exists doctors should always err on the side of preserving
life. While there may not always be hope where there is
life, there are usually more options. Indeed, in this
instance, after he is well again the patient can, if he
wishes, commit suicide.

The patient with end stage renal disease presents a
different problem. We allow him to refuse treatment and,
thus, die because in his knowledge of the disease and its
treatment and in our knowledge of him acquired during his
treatment, we know his actions to be authentic. Further,
allowing him to act on his desire preserves his independence. Here it is clear that the patient is not choosing
death but rather avoiding the consequences of treatment
which to the patient means a life the living of which is un-
supportable. The issue is sharpened in the case of the terminally ill. If biological life is medicine's goal then
the patient should be kept alive as long as possible. If
the preservation of autonomy is the goal of medicine then
one must do everything possible to maintain the integrity
of the person in the face of death.

To medicine, as to mankind, death should not matter,
life matters.

References

[1]With the assistance of Nancy McKenzie. This work was
supported in part by grants from the Henry Blum Research
Fund and the Robert Wood Johnson Foundation.

[2]Gerald Dworkin. "Autonomy and Behavior Control,"
Hastings Center Report, 6 (February 1976), 23-28.

[3]Eric J. Cassell. The Healer's Art. New York:
Lippincott, 1976, 47-83.

[4]Eric J. Cassell. The Healer's Art, p. 38.

Psychosocial Factors in Coping with Dying

E. Mansell Pattison

Current interest in the "right to die" issue has focused on an over-simplified set of either-or choices. Either the doctor or the patient has the right to decide. A person decides to either live or die. Either the person makes a decision now or does not make it. This approach obscures the fact that dying is a process. Thus, there are likely to be many choices and many persons involved in the decision-making process throughout the period of dying.

This chapter presents a clinical perspective on the psychosocial processes of dying, and will focus on the multiple questions and decisions that are raised during the dying process.

I shall discuss six issues: 1. The limits to a rational approach toward dying. 2. Coping problems throughout the dying period. 3. Concerns of the dying about death. 4. Definitions of death. 5. Coping with dying throughout the life cycle. 6. Help for the dying. I propose that we embed our inquiry into the right to die within a contextual understanding of dying.

I. The Limits To A Rational Approach Toward Dying

We are asked to understand and respond to the dying person. Yet to understand another person in his life requires that we understand the same conflicts and feelings. To understand dying in others demands that we deal with dying within ourselves.

Freud (1) suggested that the unconscious does not recognize its own death, but regards itself as immortal:

"It is indeed impossible to imagine our own death; and whenever we attempt to do so, we can perceive that we are, in fact, still present as spectators."

Freud maintains that we fear the unknownness of death. On the other hand, more recent observations suggest that death anxiety does not pertain to physical death, but to the primordial feeling of helplessness and abandonment. The fear of the unknown of death is of the unknown of annihilation of self, of being, of identity. Leveton (2) describes this sense of 'ego chill' as "a shudder which comes from the sudden awareness that our nonexistence is entirely possible."

This unknown threat cannot easily be dealt with within the self. Robert Jay Lifton (3) has graphically described his personal reactions while interviewing the survivors of the Hiroshima atomic bomb. At first he was profoundly shocked and emotionally spent as he sensed his own human frail mortality, but as the interviews went on he found himself becoming detached as a scientific observer. He did not become insensitive, but found himself inexorably developing a "psychic closing off"--in order for him to function effectively as a physician and as a scientist.

This personal account by Lifton points to a critical observation: we cannot for long look at our own non-being. Becker (4) in his book Denial of Death, says that to survive the human organism must repress his sense of frailty, must submerge his awareness of mortality, and must construct a mythology of existence--which we call our mature sense of reality. To sense our own non-being is perhaps vital, but we cannot for long look directly at it. It is like the sun. We can only look directly at the sun for a few fleeting, blinding moments at one time. For the most part, we look at the sun indirectly in the same fashion we look at our own non-being indirectly.

What is the practical import here? To talk to, work with, and understand the dying person evokes intense personal feelings. As Weisman (5) notes, the care of the dying arouses some of the most pervasive fears of all men--extinction, helplessness, abandonment, disfigurement, and loss of self-esteem. We could not long survive, much less serve our fellow man if we had to struggle continuously at the raw edge of our own existence.

There is a psychic distance to be achieved by means of compassionate detachment. Appropriate repression of our death anxieties is a necessary prelude to effective professional care. This involves the capacity to bring into consciousness the fundamental awareness of death anxiety. It means we can feel comfortable about our own finite mortality, and thus able to allow these fundamental concerns to lie out of conscious sight most of the time.

When necessary, or when evoked by life circumstance, one can then respond without major conflict to the stirrings of one's own concerns about death.

Our own attitudes toward the dying are a combination of positives and negatives. So too for the dying person, his family, relatives, and friends, and all staff. It is unrealistic to expect only positive attitudes in ourselves or in others. Some times we will be angered and frustrated by the dying. The situation of dying does not suddenly make people nice! Dying people run the gamut of all types of human beings, some likeable, some not. Some people are easy to relate to, others not. Some dying persons we will feel like helping, others not. The death of some people will cause us sorrow, others who die will provide a sense of relief, or maybe even vindictive feelings of satisfaction! It is our task to identify and assimilate all these feelings in ourselves and others, to establish a pattern of acceptance of all such feelings, to recognize that this range of emotions is part of the human experience, to integrate both positive and negative feelings, and finally, not to act upon raw emotion, but to act in accord with responsible integrity to ourselves and the dying.

We need to establish and maintain an ethical attitude that places our professional responsibility in perspective (6). We cannot be perfect. We can and will make mistakes. But we do need to try to do a decent job to the best of our ability. Maurice Levine (7) presents a practical clinical set of injunctions: 1. To avoid hostile reactions that harm the patient. 2. To avoid self-aggrandizement that may lead to operations or treatments for which one is not prepared. 3. To avoid sexually distorted attitudes that lead to possible sexually-evoked rejections or seduction of the patient. 4. To avoid revealing the confidences of patients for the sake of gossip, or to appear important in the eyes of one's spouse, friends, or colleagues. 5. To avoid excessive therapeutic ambition that leads to unnecessary procedures. 6. To avoid unnecessary stimulation of anxiety in the patient.

Mixed feelings of love and hate are universal in human relations. No important person fails to disappoint and frustrate us. The very depth of loving importance increases the probability of disappointment. For the most part we accept and tolerate the negative emotions, and tend to experience in our consciousness only the positive emotions. But it is clear that all of us harbor love and hate together. Our capacity to accept, tolerate, and even utilize the ambivalence of our feelings is one major hallmark of emotional maturity.

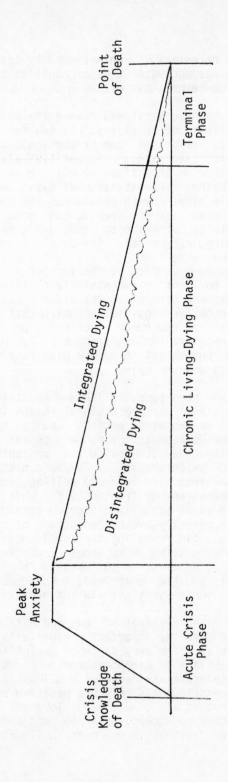

Figure 1

THE DYING TRAJECTORY

This sort of ambivalence is very much part of our attitude toward the dying. The dying person who is important to us, evokes not only feelings of tender loving compassion, but also feelings of anger, despair, frustration, disappointment, yes even hatred. If we expect only loving feelings for the dying, we shall delude ourselves, and fail to appropriately cope with the arousal of feelings of hatred.

The process of appropriate grief and mourning revolves around the successful recognition and integration of our love of and hatred toward the dead person we mourn. Similarly our attitudes toward the dying are rooted in our attitudes toward ourselves and toward others: an integration of the likeable and the despicable.

In conclusion, dying is one of the profound experiences of human life and relationships. To experience dying, either in oneself or in others, evokes the most basic emotions and conflicts of the human personality. Therefore, responsible decision-making by and for the dying is likely to be vulnerable to emotional distortions, unless we integrate both our rational thought and our sometimes irrational feelings.

II. Coping Problems Throughout The Dying Period

Death itself is not a problem of life, for death is not amenable to treatment or intervention. We may consider death only as an issue between man and God. But the process of dying may be a considerable part of a person's life. Advances in medical technology now make it possible to prolong the period of dying, so that dying may stretch over days, weeks, months, even years. For perhaps the first time in history we have many people who experience a new phase of life-the living-dying interval.

The Living-Dying Interval

All of us live with the potential for death at any moment. All of us project ahead a trajectory of our life. That is, we anticipate a certain life span within which we arrange our activities and plan our lives. And then abruptly we may be confronted with a crisis- the crisis of knowledge of death. Whether by illness or accident our potential trajectory is suddenly changed. We find that we shall die in days, weeks, months, or several years. Our life has been foreshortened. Our activities must be rearranged. We cannot plan for the potential, we must deal with the actual. It is then the period between the "crisis knowledge of death" and the "point of death" that is the living-dying interval. (This is shown in Figure 1)

The period of living-dying can be conveniently divided into three clinical phases. 1) the acute crisis phase, 2) the chronic living-dying phase, 3) the terminal phase. We can respond to the acute phase in terms of crisis intervention, so that it does not result in a chaotic disintegration of the person's life during the rest of the living-dying interval. The second task is to respond to on-going adaptive issues of the chronic living-dying phase. The third task is to assist the patient to move into the terminal phase when it becomes appropriate.

Dying Trajectories

The phases of dying are related to several different types of trajectories or "death expectations" that are set up by the crisis of knowledge of death. Glaser and Straus (8,9,10) suggest four different trajectories. 1) Certain death at a known time. In this trajectory it is possible to move rapidly from the acute phase to the chronic phase, because the time frame for resolving dying issues is quite clear. In very rapid trajectories, such as in acute leukemias or accidents, the dying process may remain only within the acute phase. 2) Certain death at an unknown time. This is a typical trajectory of chronic fatal illness. Here the problems tend to center on the maintenance of effective living in an ambiguous and uncertain time frame. 3) Uncertain death, but a known time when the question will be resolved. One example here is the radical surgery, where a successful outcome is unknown.   Thus, the patient and family may live through a continuing period of acute crisis. On the other hand, there are long-term problems, such as possible arrest of cancer, where ambiguity may remain for years. 4) Uncertain death, and an unknown time when the question will be resolved. Examples are multiple sclerosis and genetic dis - eases that leave the person facing a life of ambiguity.

Let us examine the impact of these trajectories on the dying person. First, certain trajectories are easier to cope with than uncertain trajectories. Ambiguity is always difficult to manage in life. Anxiety is generated by ambiguity and uncertainty. On the other hand, although the certainty of death may not be good news, one can plan for the specific fact of death at a known time. Thus, trajectory 1 (certain; known time) provides the dying person and the people around him a relatively specific time-frame in which to order responses. The time of most acute anxiety for the dying person is in the initial acute phase of dying when the uncertainty of events is highest. While as the certainty of exact time of death increases, anxiety diminishes.

Trajectory 3 (uncertain; known time) is somewhat similar. Here there may be prolonged anxiety in an acute phase of uncertainty--waiting for the pathology report after surgery, waiting to see if the organ transplant will work, waiting to see if the severely injured person will survive, waiting to see if the malformed infant will survive. In all of these instances, the dying trajectory is suspended in space, for no actions can be taken while the expectation is in doubt. Here the person and/or the family and staff may entertain high hopes and a positive expectation. It is understandable, then, that here there may be sudden disappointment, and frustrated anger when the hopeful expectation is suddenly dashed by the fact that the person does have a fatal diagnosis, or the illness does not respond to treatment, or the patient suddenly deteriorates and dies. Consequently, this trajectory is likely fraught with intense emotion for all envolved.

Trajectory 2 (certain; unknown time) where there is an uncertain time of death is most characteristic of chronic fatal illness. Here there is certainty of death, but the living-dying interval may stretch out over several years. It is clear that here we have prolonged emotional stress for the dying person and for the family. They live with dying. To follow the principle of certainty, the lesson here seems to be the importance of focusing on what is certain. Since the exact time of death cannot be reasonably predicted, it is important here to shift the focus to predictable daily issues of life. Thus, the dying person can live on a predictable day by day basis. Whereas in the acute trajectories one is faced with the imminent expectation of death, in this chronic trajectory, it is important to shift the focus from death per se, to the issues of living while dying.

Trajectory 4 (uncertain; unknown time) appears to be the most problematic for death itself is an uncertainty and it is ambiguous as to when the issue will be resolved. On the other hand this overall uncertainty seems to breed a high degree of anxiety that cannot be resolved, leading to dysfunctional defenses and hypochrondriacal fixation in one's physical state. Examples are multiple sclerosis and hemodialysis.

On the other hand, where medical technology has produced means of management of uncertain illness, it would appear that at least younger patients are able to make a successful adaptation.In fact, they may perceive a "reprieve from death" in their chronic stable condition. This is illustrated in cases of hemophilia, and cardiac pacemakers.

Overall, different trajectories require different coping mechanisms and vary in their evocation of anxiety and stress.

Denial and Openness

Ten years ago a common question was: Should we tell the patient or keep it a secret? Yet the care of the dying does not revolve around telling or not telling, but rather the whole panorama of human interactions that surround the dying person.

There are many levels of communication between people, and many degrees of awareness. For example, the acutely ill patient who is barely conscious should not be subjected to long discussions about the severity of his illness. He knows he is ill and may well die. Care and comfort are foremost. On the other hand, a patient who is experiencing progressive physical deterioration and is told there is nothing to worry about, may say nothing but wonder much.

It is difficult to keep secrets. The problem is when our actions say one thing and our words another.

The questions which a patient has are many. "Am I going to die?" is only the first of many questions that the patient may well need to pose and to have specific answers, not only from the physician, but from many people around him. To avoid questions about death means that one must also avoid all other questions about his life which the patient has. Kalish (11) has listed a variety of ways a patient may learn about his condition:

1. direct statements from the physician
2. overheard comments of the physician to others
3. direct statements from other personnel, including aids, nurses, technologists
4. overheard comments by staff to each other
5. direct statements from family, friends, clergy, lawyer
6. changes in the behavior of others toward the patient
7. changes in the medical care routines, procedures, medications
8. changes in physical location
9. self-diagnosis, including reading of medical books, records, and charts.
10. signals from the body and changes in physical status

11. altered response by others toward the future

It is evident that the dying person is engaged in multiple communications with many people. If the messages are congruent, the dying person can make sense out of his experience. But if the messages are confused, ambiguous, contradictory, the result is additional apprehension, anxiety, and the preventing of appropriate actions on the part of both the dying person and those around him.

Human communication is full of nuances. We should not expect that suddenly when it comes to discussions with the dying, all of our patterns of human communication should change. If we are able to talk with people about their lives in many ways comfortable and accepting to them and to us then we should be able to talk about dying in many ways that are acceptable and comfortable. Thus, I am concerned that there be opportunity, availability, and possibility for open communication with the dying.

III. Concerns Of The Dying About Death

I find that there is now rather strong unanimity among thanatologists that death itself is not a primary issue for the dying. Rather, there are many specific fears about:

1. Fear of the unknown
2. Fear of loneliness
3. Fear of sorrow
4. Fear of loss of body
5. Fear of loss of self-control
6. Fear of suffering and pain
7. Fear of loss of identity
8. Fear of regression

As the dying person looks forward on his dying trajectory he may fear the fact that he does not know what lies ahead. It is important to separate apart those things which can be known from those for which there is no answer. Diggory and Rothman (12) suggest the following fears of the unknown:

1. What life experiences will I not be able to have?
2. What is my fate in the hereafter?
3. What will happen to my body after death?
4. What will happen to my survivors?
5. How will my family and friends respond to my dying?
6. What will happen to my life plans and projects?
7. What changes will occur in my body?
8. What will be my emotional reactions?

It is evident that some of the above questions can be answered rather well immediately, some answers will be found

Figure 2

TYPES OF DEATH SEQUENCES

1.   Ideal Proximity   (note termination of hope)

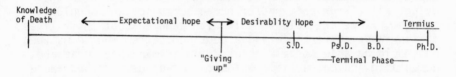

2.   Social Rejection of Patient

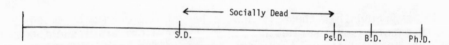

3.   Social and Patient Rejection of Death

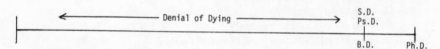

4.   Patient Rejection of Life

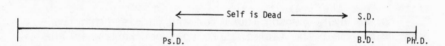

5.   Social Rejection of Death with Artificial Maintenance

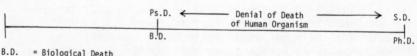

B.D. = Biological Death
Ph.D. = Physiological Death
Ps.D. = Psychic Death
S.D. = Sociological Death

in the process of time, and some cannot be answered. The issue is summed up rather well in the ancient prayer of serenity:

> "Grant me the serenity to accept the things I cannot change, the courage to change the things I can, and the wisdom to know the difference."

In sum, the decisions of the dying are for the most part about the quality of their remaining life.

IV. Definitions of Death

It might appear that the definition of death is relatively simple and poses only a technical problem of precise delineation. However, I should like to suggest four different kinds of death. In times past these four kinds of death would coalesce as a person approached terminality. However, many modern events have tended to disrupt this coalescence. (See Figure 2)

First is social death, that is, the withdrawal and separation from the patient by others. This may occur days or weeks before terminus if the patient is left alone to die. The person is treated as if dead. Some families desert the aged in nursing homes, where they may live as if dead for several years. Second is psychic death. Here the person accepts his death and regresses into himself. Such psychic death may accompany the appropriate loss of body function. But anomalies can occur, psychic death can precede terminus as in voodoo death, or in patients who predict their own death and refuse to continue living. Third is biological death. Here the organism as a human entity ceases to exist. There is no consciousness, nor awareness, such as in irreversible coma. The heart and lungs may function with artificial support but the biological organism as a self-sustaining entity is dead. Fourth is physiological death, where vital organs such as lungs, heart, and brain no longer function.

The importance of these four kinds of death is that they can occur out of phase with each other. And that becomes a major source of ethical and personal confusion. As the person enters the terminal phase, this can be considered as the onset of giving up and withdrawal. Social death would be allowing the dying person to withdraw, leading to psychic death, which is usually shortly followed by biological and then physiological death.

However, there are variations of this process. Where there is social rejection of the patient, he may become socially dead long before the other kinds of death occur. On the other hand, where there is social and personal rejection of the dying process, we have the problem of sudden death that is not anticipated nor dealt with. This can also occur when a patient suddenly deteriorates and dies contrary to expectation. This often precipitates a shocked reaction of all involved, because the anticipated trajectory has been upset. Another pattern is where the patient rejects life. This is usually met with social disapproval. For example, old people are not supposed to say they are ready to die, nor is the acutely ill person. We want people to want to live. In so doing, we may interfere with their own dying trajectory. And finally, there is the case of death of mind and body - the artificial preservation of life - in which there is social denial of the fact that both psychic death and biological death has occurred. This is currently a source of much medical-ethical controversy in our culture.

In summary, our task is to synchronize each death dimension so that optimally they will converge together in a appropriate fashion, rather than being disjointed and out of phase with each other.

V.   Coping With Death Throughout The Life Cycle

The stage of life profoundly influences one's sense of identity, one's sense of self, the sense of death, and thereby the decisions one makes. To begin with ego-coping, three general observations can be made.

First, everyone involved with dying experiences high degrees of stress. Well-seasoned medical and mental health staff do not respond with aplomb, but exhibit anguish, pain, despair, anger, fear.

Second, during the acute crisis stage of dying, more primitive and immature coping mechanisms are commonly called upon. Acute crisis calls out the most primitive defense in us. We cope the best we can. And we should neither be surprised nor dismayed to see quite primitive coping styles fleetingly emerge during acute crisis. For the most part, the dying person and his family quickly discard these primitive responses, and move on to more mature coping mechanisms. Our concern should not just be for the moment, but whether the dying person is able to move on to more adaptive mechanisms after the acute crisis has passed.

Third, we must not forget that the living-dying interval
is a time of repetitive stress. The dying person is also
physically sick, and that drains his psychic energy. While
the healthy person may effectively use many coping mechanisms,
the range becomes limited for the sick or dying person. For
example, because of physical disability, the dying person may
not be able to engage in physical activities such as recrea-
tion or work, or even such simple pursuits as conversation or
reading. Hence, the dying experience limits the repertoire
of coping mechanisms available to a person.

Ego-Coping Throughout The Life Cycle

In my book The Experience of Dying, (13) I have analyzed
the types of ego-coping mechanisms used in each life stage.
In Figure 3 I have listed these in a hierarchial sequence:
primitive, immature, neurotic, mature. There follows in the
figure, the frequency of observed coping mechanisms used by
the dying in each stage of life cycle. Again, I wish to
caution that at any given time, we may observe most of the
ego-coping mechanisms being used in transient fashion. What
we are trying to determine, however, are the more typical
coping mechanisms which the dying person uses.

First, the dying use the ego-coping mechanisms along a
developmental sequence. The youngest children only have the
most primitive coping mechanisms available. In each later
stage of life, the dying person will typically use more advanced ego-coping mechanisms, and tend to rely less on earlier types of coping. The aged generally have moved to rather mature coping mechanisms.

In early childhood we can observe the dying process
evoke primitive coping, including delusional thought, per-
ceptual distortions, and gross denial of reality. This is
not psychosis. Rather, it is the transient use of primitive
defenses. This appears to extend into the pre-school years,
but does not typically appear thereafter.

In the school age child, we see the emergent use of immature coping mechanisms. In particular the child deals with
the dying stress through externalization mechanisms. This
is of course typical of how the school age child deals with
stress and anxiety anyway.

In the adolescent, we see the appearance of the use of
intellectual coping styles as a dominant pattern, although
immature mechanisms are not abandoned. Some mature mechanisms also come in to play, especially those of intellectual
type.

FIGURE 3.

Typical Ego Coping Mechanisms
of the Dying Throughout the Life Cycle

EGO COPING MECHANISMS	EARLY CHILDHOOD	SCHOOL AGE CHILD	ADOLESCENCE	YOUNG ADULT	MIDDLE AGE	AGED
LEVEL 1. PRIMITIVE						
Delusions	+	+				
Perceptual Hallucination	+	+				
Depersonalization	+	+				
Reality Distorting Denial	+	+				
LEVEL 2. IMMATURE						
Projection	++	+++	+		+	
Denial through fantasy	++	+	+			
Hypochondriasis		++	++	++	++	++
Passive-aggressiveness		+++	++	+++	++	++
Acting-out Behavior		+++	++	+++	++	++
LEVEL 3. NEUROTIC						
Intellectualization			+++	+	+++	+
Displacement			++	++	+	
Reaction Formation			++	+++	++	
Emotional Dissociation			+++	+	+	+
LEVEL 4. MATURE						
Altruism			+		+	++
Humor			+	+	+	+
Suppression			++	+++	+++	+
Anticipatory thought			+++	+++	+++	+++
Sublimation			+	+	++	++

+   = occasional use
++   = moderate use
+++   = frequent use

In the young adult there appears a wider variety of coping mechanisms. It would seem that more immature mechanisms crop up in young adulthood. Adolescents appear to gain strength and coping ability from their parents and other adult figures. Whereas the young adult may be making the transition to independence, and thus dying comes at a particularly vulnerable time that calls forth more immature mechanisms. In the middle-aged we observe the emergence of many mature mechanisms, and less use of the immature mechanisms seen in the young adult. In the aged, although hypochrondriasis is a feature, the presence of predominantly mature coping mechanisms is manifest.

Finally, I want to reiterate that I have summarized typical coping mechanisms during the living dying interval. As noted before, the initial acute crisis phase is likely to be marked by transient maladaptive coping mechanisms. In the above analysis, I have been concerned with the chronic living-dying interval. Finally, when we come to the terminal phase of dying, we may expect the typical coping mechanisms to recede, and be replaced by isolating mechanisms, withdrawal, and increasing detachment. This withdrawal may be misinterpreted as depression. No doubt there is some depression present; our task however may not be to draw the person back into involvement with life, but rather allow them to appropriately withdraw from life.

In summary, during the dying process people do not suddenly develop new styles of coping. Rather they tend to cope with dying as they have typically coped throughout their life.

VI. Help For The Dying

To set the dying process in perspective, I should like to set forth four precepts about help for those who are dying.

First, dying is not a pathological problem that should be "treated." Thus, I do not want to present a set of "treatment plans" for the dying. It would be more accurate to consider how we "respond" to, "relate to," or "interact" with the dying.

Second, helping is a normal everyday response of human relationship; it is not something special. All of us maintain a relative stability in life because of the helping interaction with people around us. The once popular song by the Beatles says: "I get along with a little help from my friends." Helping is the corrective, supportive, inquisitive, challenging, accepting, give-and-take that comprises our valued interaction with others.

Third, helping is both doing and being. In our anxiety to accomplish something, to do something about dying, to feel we are valuable, whatever, there is zealousness to do things. But this may be for our own benefit, not for the dying. To comfort is to share. To share is the willingness to be, without having to do.

Fourth, helping with dying is the opposite of the usual sorts of helping. Usually we help people to move toward fuller engagement of life. Dying people have to be helped to disengage from life.

In working with the dying person, there is no ideal pattern, yet there are some general principles for integration of dying into the person's life style. Weisman (5) describes this as an "appropriate death." We seek to assist the dying person to live out his dying in a manner consonant with his own pattern of coping mechanisms, his own definition of the meaning of death, and his own context of values.

Following Weisman, I propose the following criteria of an "appropriate" manner of dying.

1. The person is able to face and resolve the initial crisis of acute anxiety without disintegration,

2. The person is able to reconcile the reality of his life as it is to his ego-ideal image of his life as he wanted it to be.

3. The person is able to preserve or restore the continuity of his important relationship during the living-dying interval and gradually achieve separation from his loved ones as death approaches.

4. The person is able to reasonably experience the emergence of basic instincts, wishes, and fantasies, that lead without undue conflict to gradual withdrawal and the final acceptance of death.

A second principle involves the maintenance of responses appropriate to each phase of dying. Different emotional issues and reality factors face the dying person in each of three phases of dying. Each phase calls for a different style of response. In the initial acute crisis phase he is faced with the issue of acute anxiety, and perhape high ambiguity. In the chronic living-dying phase he is faced with reality issues and coping with problems in daily living. In the terminal phase he is in need of support for achieving separation and withdrawal.

A third principle involves the terminal phase. The dying person should be helped to achieve relative <u>synchrony</u>, so that the social, psychological, physiological and biological dimensions of death tend to merge together in a coherent fashion. This means that we must attempt to maintain social and psychological attitudes that are consistent with the physiological state of the dying person.

VII. Summary

The capacity of the dying to engage in decisions about their life vary with their stage in the life cycle, their personal views and understanding of death, their available coping mechanisms, and the specific phase of the dying process. Decisions are multiple throughout the dying period. Decisions need to be made in terms of the specific values and life style of the dying person, rather than just by general principles alone.

In the history of human culture we have rarely left people to fend for themselves when faced with dying. The dying person is usually involved with many persons throughout the dying period, including family, relatives, friends, and various professionals. Therefore decisions about the dying should not be unilateral, and for the most part cannot be made by the dying person alone nor by any other one person. Dying is a complex process involving multiple decisions, decisions that need constant re-evaluation, and the greatest possible participation on the part of all concerned.

References

1.   Freud, S. Thoughts for the times on war and death. Collected papers, Vol. 4. London: Hogarth, 1915.

2.   Leveton, A. Time, death, and the ego-chill. J. Existentialism 6:69-80, 1965.

3.   Lifton, R.J. On death and death symbolism: The Hiroshima disaster. Psychiatry 27:191-210, 1964.

4.   Becker, E. The Denial of Death. New York: Macmillan, 1973.

5.   Weisman, A.D. Misgivings and misconceptions in psychiatric care of the terminal patient. Psychiatry 33:67-81, 1970.

6.   Pattison, E.M. Psychosocial and religious aspects of medical ethics. In: To Live and to Die: When, Why, and How. R.H. Williams (ed) New York: Springer-Verlag, 1973.

7.   Levine, M. The Hippocratic oath in modern dress. Cincinnati Med. J. 29:257-262, 1948.

8.   Glaser, B.G. and Straus, A.L. Awareness of Dying. Chicago: Aldine, 1966.

9.   Glaser, B.G. and Strauss, A.L. Time for Dying. Chicago: Aldine, 1968.

10. Straus, A.L. & Glaser, B.G. Anguish: A Case History of a Dying Trajectory. Mill Valley, Ca.: The Sociology Press, 1970.

11. Kalish, R.A. The onset of the dying process. Omega 1:57-69, 1970.

12. Diggory, J.C. and Rothman, D.Z. Values destroyed by death. J. Abn. Soc. Psychol. 63:205-210, 1961.

13. Pattison, E.M. The Experience of Dying. Englewood Cliffs, N.J. Prentice-Hall, 1976.

4

Strategic Relationships in Dying

Thomas C. Schelling

Ten years ago I had occasion to address the question, What is it worth to save a life? Many expensive government programs have as their purpose, or include among their consequences, the saving of lives. But except for dramatic rescues, most programs that save lives do so by reducing some statistical likelihood of death among some part of the population. Deaths are reduced in the aggregate, but we may never know who would have died, but didn't, because of some improvement in safety or reduction in risk. Even when it is known afterward whose death was averted, it wasn't known when the program was decided on who the beneficiaries would be.

Not knowing yet who will benefit, perhaps never knowing who did benefit, we can approach the issues less dramatically and more straightforwardly. It is distasteful to count costs when deciding whether a rescue crew should keep drilling in a collapsed mine where it is known there are survivors; but it is easy to count costs, and we always do, in deciding whether to install traffic lights, to take the sulfur out of the coal we burn, or to enlarge the local fire department.

Not knowing who it is that may benefit from a statistically life-saving or mortality-reducing expenditure changes the decision in another way. When we decide what it is worth to save a particular life, the life is always somebody else's. But when we reduce in small measure some widespread risk to the population--reducing air pollution or producing a flu vaccine--we who discuss the "value" of the lifesaving, even those among us who participate in the decision, are part of the population at risk. We are not ourselves immortal; we are all consumers when risks are reduced and life expectancy lengthened. We cannot confine ourselves to the moralistic question, What is it worth to us to extend some-

body else's life expectancy, or even to the legislative question, How much should some be taxed that others may have
their life expectancies lengthened? Instead we share the
question, What is it worth to us to reduce the risks that
afflict us, to increase our life expectancy, to save some
among us—we've no way of knowing whom—that might otherwise
die? There is nothing inspirational in deciding whether it
is worth the cost to install a lightning rod on the roof of
my own house; and there is nothing wrong with self-interest
in voting on whether to increase my town's expenditure on
libraries, tennis courts, traffic controls or fire equipment.

This question, What is it worth to me to reduce the
risks to my own life, or what is it worth to my family to
reduce the risks to my family, is not the only point of view
from which to enlighten the issues involved in public programs to save lives. But it is one point of view, an important one, sometimes the right one, and a refreshing check on
the valuations one may arrive at by supposing vicariously
that it is always "they" who die and "we" who make the decisions.

For what I wrote ten years ago I chose as title the
familiar slogan, "The Life You Save May Be Your Own." In
this symposium I want the reader to join me in supposing
that the "right to die" we are talking about is our right,
not somebody else's. Most of the people who deal professionally with the subject, including some contributing to
this volume, are professionally concerned with the dying—
ministering to them, defending their rights, providing them
help or protection, designing institutions for their comfort
and dignity. I do not professionally deal with the dying;
I do not represent them or advise them or treat them, nor
do I deal with their families or their physicians or their
attorneys, or their hospitals and nursing homes. I also am
not myself dying, as far as I know; so I do not speak for
"them" nor do I have a particular plea on behalf of a particular group of victims.

I merely represent the consumer. I am somebody who,
like everybody else, is going to die. Like most of us I am
going to die but I do not know how or in what circumstances,
whether suddenly or after protracted illness, conscious or
unknowing, expensively or cheaply, mute or articulate, in
dignity or defilement, a comfort or a burden to my family or
without any family at all.

And I ask myself what institutional arrangements I
would like to govern my dying. What rules or traditions or
practices would I like to be established? What rights and

privileges and obligations would I like to govern my dying
and the dying of others, recognizing that I shall share in
the expense of the things that cost money, that I shall
share in obligations to the dying just as I enjoy the obligations of others when I am the dying, and that the claims
I would like to make when it is my turn to die will be the
claims that the dying make on me when I am not yet dying?

From this point of view the issue is not the asymetri-
cal one of my moral obligation to the dying, or their moral
obligations to us, or what I shall want from you when it is
my turn to be the dying. It is the more practical ques-
tion--terribly important, but properly self-centered--of the
arrangements for dying under which I would prefer to live
and die.

For concreteness let me suppose that the various legal,
ethical, financial and professional arrangements that govern
dying were determined within the individual states and that
each among the 50 states had different traditions and practices and laws and institutions with respect to dying and
death. Suppose that different states have different "rights
to die" and "rights to live," different divisions of authority among physicians, hospital directors, public officials,
spouses and parents and guardians, different ways to allo-
cate scarce medical resources or to apportion the costs of
caring for the dying, different rules of privacy and immunity, different laws about suicide and malpractice and insur-
ance claims, different rules for clergy, ombudsmen, and the
judiciary. In which state would I prefer to live and die?

Having invited you to look at the issues from this
standpoint I am now going to disappoint you. This may be
the right way to look at the subject, or at least one useful way, but it is not one that makes the subject any easier. From this point of view the subject is less loaded with
morality, duty, and right and wrong; but it may be intellectually easier to identify one's duty in a particular
situation than to identify that complex of rights and obligations with which one would choose to surround oneself if
one had to do the choosing.

But a few of the issues do become a little easier to
manage from this point of view. First, we can now disagree,
even disagree sharply, about the regimes for dying that we
prefer, without having to acknowledge that if one of us is
right the other must be wrong, and especially without having
to conclude that if one of us is morally correct the other
must be morally wrong. Those among us who can differ about
the lifestyles we choose but who can respect each other be-

cause lifestyle is a matter of taste, may now differ in the
deathstyles we prefer. The way of dying that appeals to me
may not be the one that appeals to you but, then, ways of
living that appeal to me may not appeal to you. The amenities that I would sacrifice to avoid discomfort at dying may
not be the amenities that you would sacrifice to avoid particular discomforts at dying, but then we differ about the
trades we make every day in where and how we live and work
and divide our time between earning money and enjoying lei-
sure, or the way we trade sociability for solitude. So in
choosing, from the point of view of dying, the state we want
to live in, there is no need to feel that anything fundamental is necessarily wrong if we choose differently among the
states.

The consumer point of view is also helpful in thinking
about how great the sacrifices are that we should want to
make for the dying, or to keep people from dying, and what
the limits are to the time and trouble and money we should
devote to the dying and to those who may die. Because from
this point of view it is not what we owe them and ought to
do for them, or what others owe us and ought to do for us;
it is where we would choose to set the balance when it is
both our time and trouble and money when they are dying, and
their time and trouble and money when we are dying. The
question is what bargain I want to make. How far do I want
to impair my joy in living to relieve the discomfort of dying? How much do I want to be obliged to help others in
their distress so that they are obliged to help me in mine?
How much of the burden of my dying do I want others to accept
if I must in like measure share the burden of their dying?

To withhold anything that might prolong a comfortable
life may seem a dereliction when viewed unilaterally, and
give rise to feelings of guilt; but to agree ahead of time
that you don't have to do it for me if I don't have to do it
for you may be a sensible bargain. If I choose a regime in
which a spouse is not to be indefinitely enslaved to a helpless partner, you cannot easily dismiss me as heartless and
selfish if we don't yet know which of the two partners I am
going to be.

This question of the "rights of the dying" is different
from that of the "right to die," but they are related. The
right to die is occasionally the right to relieve loved ones
of a physical and financial and emotional burden; and the
"right to die" may include the right to relinquish certain
claims for living that, viewed as reciprocal obligations,
make a poor bargain.

But to recognize this principle does not mean it can be implemented. Let me go back to that question of saving lives with which I opened this essay. They who go to sea in boats may all agree that it is uneconomical to search more than one day for somebody lost at sea. While further search is not hopeless and people are occasionally rescued after the first day's effort, it is enormously expensive; and they who stand to benefit have to pay the cost of trying to rescue each other, and find it a cost not worth paying. Having agreed to that, you are lost at sea and at the end of a day we haven't found you. It will not be easy to curtail the rescue. Especially if the community is small and we know you and must live with the thought that had we tried one more day we might have saved you, and if we must face your family. One more day and another and another may be irresistible, though we damn ourselves for wasting our resources, not at all reconciled by the thought that, when it is our own turn to be lost at sea, others will waste their time and money in a fruitless search for us.

But if search beyond a certain distance requires aircraft and we agree not to acquire the aircraft, we cannot mount the extra search and there will be neither guilt nor a coerced waste of resources. We took the decision together—the one who is lost having shared in the decision—and each took the decision knowing that the person lost at sea could be himself. Any agreement not to waste resources taking care of each other in extremity, however sound the bargain that it represents, will be hard to enforce unless we can deny ourselves the ability.

That situation is at one extremity of the spectrum of the "right to die." Let me divide the spectrum arbitrarily into three segments. The three correspond to the demands, "Let me die," "Help me die," and "Make me die." The third, "Make me die," involves at least two very different concepts. One is unilateral: make me die for my sake, I ought to die but can't (and can't even want to). The second is the reciprocal bargain discussed a moment ago: make me die because that's what I contracted for. This second, stronger case, not "Please make me die" but "Go ahead and make me, that's the bargain," is not what people usually have in mind in discussing rights rather than obligations. But it is worth including here because the right to be held to a bargain is usually a prerequisite to making the bargain.

The "right to be sued" for breach of contract sounds paradoxical, but if one cannot be sued for breach of contract one cannot find anybody to enter the contract. The

right to have my mortgage foreclosed is part of the right to
borrow money. The right to enter an enforceable contract is
one of those important rights that we grant to corporations
and that we withhold from children until they reach 18 or
21. If they can't repossess your car they won't sell you
the car on credit; if they can't hold you to your guarantee
they won't buy your merchandise. And the "right to forego"
excessive claims for medical support will be part of the
right to avoid excessive reciprocal obligations.

The more poignant case and more philosophically troub-
ling is the demand, "Make me die for my sake." Not "Let me"
but "Make me." Make me, despite my wish to go on living,
despite my pleading to be kept alive, despite my most desperate efforts to hang on to life. How does this situation
arise, and what are the principles we should want to govern
the response?

It arises of course when I have asked you in advance
to see that I die if certain conditions befall me and to
disregard any change of mind that the fear of imminent death
may seem to induce. I have asked you not to heed my pleas
when I become so deranged that I won't go through with it.
I have commanded you not to let me live in such condition,
and if I should become terrified of dying you must not prolong my terror.

We confront the question, Which is the authentic "I"
in that crisis? There are probably two of me, one who was
in command when I made anticipatory arrangements, contemplated the alternatives and gave my instructions and warned
you not to heed that other one who would surface and speak
with my voice when it was time to die. Is that crisis the
moment of truth or the moment of derangement?

A similar problem of authenticity arises in many contexts, though not often with quite the finality of this decision to heed or not to heed the plea to rescind the earlier instruction. Someone addicted to alcohol, drugs or
cigarettes, or a compulsive over-eater, may ask you under
no circumstances to heed a plea for a smoke or a drink or a
dose or another helping, even if he pleads or screams with
tears in his eyes. Indeed, the more frantically he pleads
the more you may be enjoined to recognize what a horror you
perpetuate, while momentarily relieving it, if you accede.
I am told that people who are determined to try parachuting
are sometimes incapable of leaping from the aircraft and
may need and want and request to be forcibly expelled in
the event they freeze at the last minute. Which is the

authentic individual, the one who grips the doorframe until
his knuckles turn white, desperately resisting the foot
against his back, or the one that said, on the ground a few
minutes earlier, to use all the strength you need to get
him out and not to mistake his phobia for himself?

I do not believe it is possible to hold your breath and
die; before you die your urge to breathe will overcome your
urge to die, however much you regret it once you've caught
your breath. If someone is to help you he must not interpret your struggle for breath as a reversal of your decision.

But these considerations do not settle the question,
they merely create it. It is profoundly important to recognize that to let somebody live who previously chose to die
can be as heartless and irresponsible as giving a second
helping to the person whose doctor prescribed diet; but how
do you know the person isn't starving, and how do you know
the one who earlier elected to die hasn't really seen at
last what he never saw before, and genuinely changed his
mind? I am arguing only for the legitimacy of the problem,
not for any particular solution.

"Let me die" at the other end of the spectrum raises
tortuous issues, even for those for whom no divine laws are
involved. Before mentioning some of the complications that
most trouble me, let me point out that the let-help-make
division is itself ambiguous: unplugging my respirator does
all three. "Let" implies that I want you to; "Make" may
imply that I shall not want you to; but the difference is
in the motive rather than the action. And the difference
between letting and helping will often depend just on what
the norm is: not removing the medicine with which I can
overdose myself is "letting" if the custom is to let me be
custodian of my own medicine, "helping" if the custom is to
keep it out of reach.

Letting me die can take a number of forms. There is
the physical one of allowing me the means to end my life;
but there is also relieving me of any moral obligation to
stay alive, or of guilt or legal sanctions, providing moral
support, helping to avert the shame or disgrace of people
to whom my death will be a reproach or a scandal.

At first glance I like the idea of being allowed to
die. It isn't asking you to become an accessory by helping;
it isn't asking you to overrule my pleas if I change my
mind. It is not a right that I exercise against you, a
claim that places a duty on you; it only asks you not to

interfere or to impose hindrance or penalty.

But some rights bring responsibilities and verge on obligations. The "right" of a 17-year-old to volunteer in wartime can subject him to a sense of obligation. The right to early retirement can be construed as an obligation to get out and clear the way for others. The right to depart this world at least raises the question whether the decent thing wouldn't be to discontinue being a burden, an annoyance, an expense and a source of anxiety to the people in whose care a dying person finds himself. My disability is a burden we share as long as no alternative is available; it is a burden of which I can relieve you if the option of dying is known to be available. And it is an option that can preoccupy us whether or not there is any immediate intention of taking advantage of it.

If I could die and relieve you of the burden and the expense, how could you persuade me you truly wanted me to live? Telling me so, repeatedly, will only demonstrate your awareness of my option, remind me of it and remind me that I cannot take it for granted. And how do you discuss it behind my back? If my surviving gains me a few years of life of exceedingly low quality, and condemns my spouse to the same when she could have been free of me had I exercised my right to go, and you feel this keenly, just how do you perceive your obligation to her, including your obligation to respect what she believes to be her obligations, and how do you mediate your obligations to her and your obligations to me? How do I manage my guilt upon awaking every morning, knowing I am spoiling another day of her life; and how do I evaluate the guilt she will feel if I take my life for her sake?

These are rhetorical questions as I pose them now, to remind us that freedom of choice is not always welcome and that more choice can mean more conflict, that rights may entail the obligation to exercise them. In the actual event they would be not rhetorical questions but real ones. I raise these unhappy questions not to suggest that they are unanswerable, and that the right to die would bring more grief than it would remove. My purpose is only to illustrate how hard it is to anticipate how much freedom we should want and what kinds of constraints and safeguards may be needed.

"Help me die" is even more laden with potential anxiety, conflict and misunderstanding, suspicion, guilt and mistrust. Help can mean anything from "Let me—just don't intervene, when intervening to stop me would be your normal

response;" to "Do it for me, I can't do it myself; without
your help I am doomed to live and suffer." And there are
at least two important ways that I can be unable to do it
for myself; I may be physically unable, or like that para-
chutist I may be unable to make myself act.

The right to your help is the right to make you an
accessory. If someone will help and someone won't, the
first appears guilty of complicity. And if you volunteer
your help--if I need your help even in raising the subject--
how am I to interpret your suggestion that, with your help,
I can accomplish my own removal? When I ask your help in
dying are you to interpret that as a plea to be talked out
of it, especially if I say I want to die to unburden others?
What witnesses shall we need to allay my fears that you may
"help me" when I don't want the help, or that you misunder-
stand me? What witnesses shall we need to protect you from
the suspicion that you were a little too ready with your
help? And if I continually change my mind, asking help in
the morning and rescinding my request in the evening, begging to live and then begging to die, which of the two is
my authentic self to whom you are responsible?

"Help" can mean many things, only one of which is being instrumental in some lethal process. It can mean comfort and moral support as I take a critical step myself.
It can mean phoning the physician or the attorney or making
legal arrangements, or helping me go where I can solve the
problem myself or find professional help for the terminal
process. It can even mean defending me from those who
would intervene to prevent my dying. Most of all it may
mean helping me to reach the right decision, whichever decision that is, sharing the anxiety and the uncertainty and
the moral burden, even while being yourself an interested
party.

The least burdensome kind of help and the least divi-
sive would probably be participation in the arrangements
we might make together, while death is still remote and
hypothetical, for a decent death in certain contingencies.
Let me propose a piece of technology out of science fiction,
which I imagine is actually feasible. A particular contingency in which many people appear willing to hope they
would die is a severely disabling stroke, a stroke that
leaves one bedridden and inarticulate. Some of us may wish
to die because of the horror and indignity of being unable
to feed ourselves and unable even to smile if we should
recognize our visitors; some of us want to remove a penalty
that no one would dream of inflicting on the family, and a

gratuitous expense for which no value is received. Now suppose there were available a diagnostic contrivance that could be implanted in the brain that, in the event of cerebral hemorrhage, would measure the severity, remaining inactive if the predicted paralysis were below some limiting value but fatally aggravating the condition above that limit. My conjecture is that the principle would be attractive to many of us.

In line with the consumer point of view that I am urging, I can also conjecture that it would be unattractive to many of us. I should be surprised, however, if even among those who would deprecate such mechanical contingent suicide, or automatic euthanasia, it wouldn't be considered superior to a contractual arrangement to provide an equivalent result by human hand.

I've said nothing about the physician's role. I doubt whether it is good to give the physician much of a role, beyond a diagnostic and analytical role, in the decisions to let or to help or to make a patient die. It must be hard enough to be a good physician without being lawyer, clergyman, ombudsman, referee and family counsellor or family arbiter, and it may help both patient and physician and their relation to each other to have the physician unambiguously devoted to the patient's life and comfort. But because the choice of treatment is often a trade of life expectancy for quality of life, the physician cannot always exempt himself from a role in the decisions to shorten or lengthen life. If the physician's role has typically been a dominant one, that may be because no other profession, at least no other lay profession, has been rash enough to seek aggressively an important role for itself.

As a consumer who is not yet a patient, I am attracted to the notion that an attorney is closer than a physician to the kind of profession that may need to be involved in exercising the right to die. It is after all attorneys who deal with many of the consequences of death, drawing wills and serving as executors when decisions must be made about the custody of children or the distribution of wealth. The issues in the right to die involve conflict of interest, enforcement of contract, and the maintenance of legal proprieties without which the whole arrangement could degenerate into something quite barbarian. Something like an ombudsman or executor may be needed, especially if that person could be chosen well in advance of the contingency, the way some of us choose the executors named in our wills.

I am not ready to choose which among 50 variegated regimes for dying I might wish to live in. If they actually existed in great diversity we should have experience that would make the choice a more informed one, perhaps an easier one. The whole subject is in dispute, but not in great enough dispute, not enough to generate widespread imaginative exploration and critical evaluation of competing alternatives.

5

The Right to Die Garrulously

Alasdair MacIntyre

I want in this paper to make two central points: one, rather more briefly, about rights and one, at somewhat greater length, about death and dying. On rights I want to distinguish three classes of claim to the possession of a right. There are first of all claims to rights where the right in question has been, or is alleged to have been, created (rather than merely recognized) by positive law, and secondly where the right in question has been, or is alleged to have been, created by a promise. With these types of claim I shall not be concerned further. The third type of claim is to a type of right alleged to belong to human beings as such, independently of what any positive law may say. Examples of such alleged rights are those cited in the Declaration of Independence and in the U.N. Declaration of Human Rights and those defended by Professor Ronald Dworkin in his recent book Taking Rights Seriously (1), including an alleged right of every human being to "equal concern and respect." (2)

It is presumably rights of this third kind that are invoked in most discussions of death and dying. The question: "Do individuals have a right in certain circumstances - for example, extreme and unrelievable pain or the occurrence of such brain damage that there can be no possibility of recovery except as an idiot - to be deprived of further life-support or to have their life taken, provided that at the relevant time they do consent or have consented to this?" is invariably discussed as a question about an alleged natural or human right which individuals as such do or do not possess. This is perhaps unfortunate, because it seems clear that the answer to all such questions must be 'No'.

This is not because of the merits or demerits of any of the particular arguments advanced about suicide or about brain damage or about medical technology. It is because there

are no such rights. The ground for asserting this is the
second best of all possible grounds for making universal negative existential assertions: nobody has ever given us the
slightest reason for believing that there are. (The best of
all possible grounds for making such an assertion is that the
concept in question necessarily has no embodiment, as e.g.
that of the greatest integer).

In the eighteenth century the existence of such natural
rights was defended on the grounds that the statements asserting them were self-evident truths; but the required concept of self-evidence could not be sustained. In the United
Nations declaration of 1949 what has since become the normal
U.N. practice of not giving reasons for <u>any</u> assertions what-
soever is followed with great rigor. And Professor Dworkin's
retort to the charge that the existence of such rights cannot
be proved is only that from the fact that a statement cannot
be demonstrated to be true, it does not follow that that
statement is not true. (<u>3</u>) Which is true, but could be used
equally in vindication of every unprovable statement whatso-
ever. Some other recent philosophers have tended to speak
here of their and our moral 'intuitions'; but one of the
things that we learn from the history of philosophy is that
the occurrence of the word 'intuition' in philosophy is usually a sign that something has gone badly wrong.

I conclude that there are no valid claims to rights of
this third kind. Such rights are at one with unicorns,
witches and Meinong's glass mountain. Jeremy Bentham said
the last word about them, philosophically if not chronologi-
cally, when he declared that 'natural rights' are 'nonsense'
and 'imprescriptible, inalienable natural rights' 'nonsense
on stilts'. But this radical conclusion does not terminate,
it only opens my present enquiry. For there are a fourth
class of claims to rights to the discussion of which we must
now turn.

In the game of chess each player has a right to move in
turn, the player who is White having the right to move first.
In natural science scientists have the right to use the find-
ings of other scientists, provided they acknowledge priority
of publication. At the coronation of the O'Neill,the
O'Cathaín had the right to place the crown on the O'Neill's
head. (<u>4</u>) In each of these cases the possession of the right
is only intelligible in the context of a developed and complex form of human practice. The exercise of such rights is
a necessary part of such practices and their violation is to
varying degrees destructive of such practice. The justification of the claim to possess such a right must initially refer

us to the rules of the practice and thereafter to the possible justifications of the practice. Notice that such rights
do not belong to individuals as such, but only to individuals
in virtue of their filling certain roles, roles the effective
discharge of which is essential to the practice. Positive
law may on occasion recognize certain of these rights or even
prescribe that they shall be enforced. But such rights are
not created by positive law in the way, for example, that the
right of a Massachusetts resident to challenge what he or she
takes to be an incorrect billing within sixty days is created
by positive law.

In order to discover whether a given claim of this fourth
type is or is not valid, it is obvious that we must first
determine whether there is or is not a practice in the relevant area of human life, understanding by a practice some
form of rule-governed behavior which has its own goods, in
the way in which games, scientific enquiry and Irish tribal
rituals do. To say this is to suggest strongly to the contemporary American mind that rights of this fourth type could
have nothing to do with any alleged right to die. For we
characteristically take it for granted that death and dying
are episodes in or terminating the lives of individuals which
are not and could not be a part of any coherent practice in
the required sense. That is, our dominant culture lacks any
coherent concept, and perhaps any concept at all, of a right
way to die or a wrong way to die, of a good death or a bad
death.

Yet in lacking such concepts and correspondingly lacking
any shared practice of death and dying, modern American culture is at odds with many other cultures, including a number
of its own predecessors: American Indian, some African,
Irish, some Asian, much of the European middle ages and some
of the ancient world. I am not going to argue in this paper
for the superiority of the perspective on death and dying of
such cultures to our contemporary American standpoint; all
that I shall be able to do is to give some account of what
this alternative perspective is.

It was Robert Herz (5), Durkheim's pupil, who first drew
the attention of anthropologists to the fact that in certain
societies - his own studies were in Indonesia - death is not
only or primarily the terminating episode in the life of an
individual, but an event in the life of that society of which
the individual formed a part and from which he drew his identity. The funeral rites are an occasion in which the social
group confronts the loss of part of itself and summons up the
resources to reconstitute itself. The dead individual is not
wholly lost to the group; as spirit or as ancestor or both he

is still part of that continuity which links the living both
to the dead and to the as yet unborn. Death and the ceremonies of death are thus a moment of transition for both the
individual and the group.

From the point of view which Herz describes, a society or
a group - a tribe, a family, a local community, a nation - is
not a collection of individuals, each with his or her own independent identity, who merely happen to be united in social
relationships. Rather the group is primary and the individual's identity is partly, but crucially constituted by his or
her membership of and place in the group. The individual who
lacks any such membership and place, who has no identity but
his own, is that marginal man "the stranger." And when a
stranger dies, there is nobody to mourn that trivial passing.
With the stranger we may make agreements or temporary arrangements for one transient purpose or another; but contractual
arrangements - those very arrangements which the theorists
who celebrated the birth of modern individualist society,
such as Hobbes and Locke, thought to underlie all social
relationships - constitute no fundamental social bond.

From the standpoint of the communities which Herz describes, modern America would appear for the most part as
merely a collectivity of strangers, of only accidentally
related individuals; and the predominant individualist attitudes to death and dying would confirm them in their view.
Yet it is not merely from the standpoint of the Malay archi-
pelago in the early twentieth century that America would
look like this. In a quite different culture, one in which
our own is rooted, Sophocles' Philoctetes describes himself
as "friendless, solitary, without a city, a corpse among the
living" (6) and the last characterization follows from the
first three. To lack the identity conferred by a city and by
friendship (in the Greek understanding of that concept) is to
be an unburied corpse. And to be an unburied corpse is to
lack that relationship to the community which is conferred by
funeral rites.

What unites these very different cultures then is a conception of death as a distinctively social event and of the
dying man and those around him as fulfilling social roles.
These roles have both a backward looking and a prospective
character. The backward-looking aspect of the role of the
dying man concerns the fact that death is the completion of
life. "Call no man happy until he is dead" said the prudent
Greek proverb; but what follows is that death is precisely
the point at which a man may be called happy. The death of
such a man is in no way to be regretted and mourning for such
a man is not a species of regret. What then is the connec-

tion between death, the completion of life and happiness?

The conception of death and dying in at least some of such societies is inseparable from a conception of life as divided into determinate stages each of which specifies a type of role. To have passed through the stages is to have reached the right time to die and it is a fundamental conviction of such societies that there is a time when it is right to die. To die before one's time is a terrible misfortune, unless one gave one's life as a sacrifice for the social group, in battle, for instance, and so completed an honorable life in another way. The right time to die may be conventionally fixed at some particular age, that of seventy, for example. But no individual is free to make a choice in this matter. The right time for him to die will come sooner or later and he must wait for it. Philippe Ariés (7) has presented convincing evidence that in such societies men possess an ability to recognize the approach of that moment, an ability that has disappeared together with the concept of there being such a moment. That there should be such an ability must seem to us in some ways strange; but it will perhaps appear less strange if we realize that the whole of life is in this perspective an approach to one's death. It is in the period before death that one becomes one of the old, that is of those who have assimilated the moral and social knowledge that has been handed down. The old preserve and enrich the tradition; their stories and sayings are the collective inherited memory of the society. Hence the young cannot afford not to listen to the old. Nor is becoming old in any way a misfortune; every period of life has its own advantages and disadvantages. One of the disadvantages of being young is that one necessarily lacks what only the old can teach. This is why, as Aristotle noted, the young cannot excel in moral philosophy.

Once again the contrast with contemporary America is almost too obvious. Here death is often feared and old age, if anything, is feared more. The old have no assigned respected role in the community. Their stories are treated not as inherited wisdom, but as boring anecdotes. A whole mythology about the declining powers of the old has been constructed. The old have become functionless, just as the dying have no socially recognized role.

This deprivation of role and function is clearly connected to another difference between America and the type of traditional society which I am trying to characterize. The old in that type of society are those who make the present one with the past. But the past in America is the object of ambiguity and suspicion. History has for some considerable

time been the least popular subject in American high schools.
Apart from a few patriotic episodes, there is little or no
shared social memory. This does not of course mean that the
past, American European and African, is not as omnipresent in
America as elsewhere. Fragmented traditions and mythologies
draw all the more power from the fact that their very existence, let alone their power, goes so largely unrecognized.
But the power of the past in the present has in our culture
been divorced from explicit social function; and so unsur-
prisingly any conception of death as the moment at which we
become one with the past has been lost too.

The role of the dying man is therefore twofold in the
relevant type of traditional society. On the one hand he has
to make that reckoning with his own past life which is required, if life is to be completed satisfactorily, if his
life is to be called happy: debts must be paid, sins must be
confessed, farewells must be made, each with the appropriate
ceremony. If we owe a cock to Aesculapius, we must pay it.
But at the same time the dying man has to hand on to the next
generation or generations the tasks and the possessions that
have hitherto been his. He must tell them now what he will
never be able to tell them again. Hence the symbolic importance of the deathbed scene. The dying man has both a duty
and a right to speak at that point at whatever length he
chooses. He has the right to die garrulously.

This role and function can like any other be discharged
well or badly. The dying man owes it to others to perform it
and to perform it well. It is in the context of these observations that the question of a right to die can be raised
once more. What from the perspective of this kind of alien
culture would have to be said about such a right? Part of
the answer is clear. If there is a right time to die, and a
time which it is not open to one to choose, then one can have
no right to bring about one's own death prematurely. If one
owes participation in the ceremonies of death to others, then
once again one can have no right to deprive them or indeed
oneself of those ceremonies. Hence there can be no general
right to suicide.

It is a good deal more difficult to pose the question of
how in the perspective afforded by such cultures one would
have to argue about the type of case in which either consciousness has been disintegrated or shortly will be by ex-
tremes of pain perhaps combined with the effects of certain
drugs or consciousness has been lost altogether because of
brain-damage, but life can still be maintained by the expensive resources of modern medical technology or consciousness,
but only idiot consciousness, can be restored after such

brain-damage. For it is characteristic of such traditional
societies that they tend to disappear early under the impact
of just those technologies and economic forms which in the
end produce the contemporary dilemmas of medical ethics.
Hence any discussion of how they might have responded is
bound to be speculative.

One thing however is clear. In all these conditions
physical death has been disjoined from any possible role for
the dying man. The tasks which such traditional cultures
assigned to the role of the dying man cannot be discharged
well or badly for they cannot be discharged. Hence in such
cases all those reasons which led us to conclude that there
could be no general right to suicide have no application.
Hence there is no reason to conclude that the patient has not
in such circumstances a right to die. Anyone therefore whose
premises derived from this cultural tradition would perhaps
have to reach conclusions at odds <u>both</u> with those contemporary conservative moralists, often though not always Roman
Catholic, who argue that because suicide is wrong there can
be no such right to die <u>and</u> with those contemporary liberal
moralists, often though not always Protestants or secularists,
who argue for the existence of such a right on the basis of a
view that suicide is a permissible type of act.

I said earlier that I was not going to argue for or
against the superiority of the traditional perspective which
I have described to our contemporary American point of view.
To do so we should have to explore the rival metaphysical
presuppositions of these two alien and antagonistic forms of
human culture; for such radically different and incompatible
views of death and dying presuppose rival views of human
nature, rival accounts of the nature of morality, indeed
rival ontologies. The argument therefore would have to extend far beyond the scope of this paper. Nonetheless it will
not have escaped notice that my very mode of description presupposes a sympathetic identification with the traditional
and a certain hostility to modernity. So that one response
even to my method of posing the questions about the right to
die may be to suggest I am raising considerations interesting
enough to the antiquarian, but now socially irrelevant. After
all the cultures of which I speak have each and every one,
when they confronted modernity, been substantially defeated
by the modernization process. So that to look for the restoration of their standpoint in our own culture will seem to
many hopelessly romantic and anachronistic. The gap between
them and us seems too wide; and their standpoint, it might be
noted, is as much at odds with our humanity at its best as it
is with our inhumanity at its worst. From the standpoint of

the cultures in which a dying man's dignity derives from his
and others' sense of the tasks which he has to perform, poli-
cies of kindness towards the dying are as irrelevant as poli-
cies of neglect. Is then the metaphysical argument between
the two types of culture not even worth joining because
history has already decided the issue? Is my own standpoint
nothing but a fragment of irrelevant medievalism?

There are at least two reasons for not assenting to
these suggestions too hastily. The first is that there have
been growing signs lately of an American ability to recognize
the rootlessness of our social condition and to look for some
means of remedying that rootlessness. But I doubt if a socially shared recovery of roots is possible without altering
our socially shared attitudes to death. For a central thesis
of this paper has been that our attitudes to death and to
aging on the one hand and our attitudes to history and the
past on the other are at key points inseparable.

A second reason for those who share my point of view not
to accept so dismissive a response too easily is rather different. Our attitudes do indeed derive from the European
middle ages; but the civilization of the middle ages was itself a response to a constellation of problems not unfamiliar
in the contemporary sense. First a period in which a high
culture became the victim of a loss of literacy, of inflation
and of the growth of new forms of large-scale property; and
then an ensuing collapse into the barbarism of the Dark Ages.
Out of which the medieval world grew, relying on the strength
of that in the culture which had enabled it to survive barbarism. If then 'the middle ages' is a name which we give to
one possible outcome of barbarism, a realistic analysis of
the contemporary American scene may suggest that the middle
ages may turn out to lie in our future as well as in our past,
and not necessarily in too distant a future; for consider
another way of viewing the implications of my argument. In
the first part of the paper I rejected any concept of natural
or human rights attaching to individuals as such as intellectually untenable. But if the case against such rights is as
overwhelming as I think it is, why have they been so widely
appealed to? One central answer is that appeal to such
rights has seemed to give us a ground, a sufficient reason,
for treating with respect and care those whom we could find
no good reason for treating with respect and care in the context of our ordinary social relationships. In traditional
societies it is not hard to find such good reasons. Why
should I treat this dying person with respect and care? Because he or she is a member of my family, my community, my
tribe. What if he or she is not? Then I must treat this

stranger as a member of my family, my community, my tribe, as
my neighbor. But what happens when those of my family, community, tribe or whatever are weakened and attenuated as they
are in the modernization process? When there is no set of
social relationships which define what it is to be a neighbor?
Then the only resort is to appeal to me to show respect and
care for the suffering or dying stranger <u>because he is a
human being</u>. But if his claim to consideration arises only
from his being a man, then it must be because some set of
rights attaches to <u>being a human being</u>. And in this case
everybody must have rights. Or so I reconstruct an argument
implicit in modern appeals to rights, functioning to fill a
social void, and relying on its kinship to unacknowledged
older notions, both religious and legal, for part of its
power.

Abstract humanity, however, turns out to be a relatively
impotent moral notion and appeals to human rights as such
have in the past only functioned effectively in their negative form. "You have no right to do this to us ....." ad-
dressed by the spokesmen of suffering communities to their
oppressors - whether by Massachusetts colonists to King George
III or by Robespierre to those who would limit the suffrage
in revolutionary France or by black people in Alabama and
Mississippi to the post-Reconstruction South - can be a crucial form of political expression which does not suffer from
any of the intellectual defects of the positive argument for
natural rights; indeed it is precisely because of the fatal
defects in the positive argument that it is able to make its
case. If there are no human rights as such, then no human
being can have a natural right to oppress another. So it is
easy to understand why the appeal to natural rights has been
historically powerful as protest or as revolution, but not as
a ground for individual caring and concern for other individuals, such as the dying and the incurable.

I am suggesting, then, that in a society dominated by the
concepts of abstract individualism the problems of the dying
and the incurable may to some large extent be insoluble; but
from this it does not follow that there is no ground for hope.
It is rather to suggest that, to the extent that we do
grapple socially and morally with the problems of the dying
and intellectually with the problem of the right to die, we
may gradually mount at the level of local communities - those
of the home and the hospital - one of the most effective
challenges that modern individualism has so far had to meet.

Footnotes

1. Ronald Dworkin, <u>Taking Rights Seriously</u>. London: Duck-
   worth, 1976.
2. <u>Op.cit.</u>, p.180.
3. <u>Op.cit.</u>, p.81.
4. Francis John Burne, <u>Irish Kings and High-Kings</u>.London:
   Batsford, 1973.
5. Robert Herz, <u>The Collective Representation of Death</u> in
   <u>Death and the Right Hand</u>. Trans. Robert & Claudia Need-
   ham. London: Cohen and West, 1960.
6. L.1018.
7. Philippe Ariés, <u>Western Attitudes Towards Death</u>. Baltimore and London: John Hopkins University Press, 1974.

Euthanasia

Philippa Foot

The widely used Shorter Oxford English Dictionary gives
three meanings for the word "euthanasia": the first, "a
quiet and easy death"; the second, "the means of procuring
this"; and the third, "the action of inducing a quiet and
easy death." It is a curious fact that no one of the three
gives an adequate definition of the word as it is usually
understood. For "euthanasia" means much more than a quiet
and easy death, or the means of procuring it, or the action
of inducing it. The definition specifies only the manner of
the death, and if this were all that was implied a murderer,
careful to drug his victim, could claim that his act was an
act of euthanasia. We find this ridiculous because we take
it for granted that in euthanasia it is death itself, not
just the manner of death, that must be kind to the one who
dies.

To see how important it is that "euthanasia" should not
be used as the dictionary definition allows it to be used,
merely to signify that a death was quiet and easy, one has
only to remember that Hitler's "euthanasia" program traded
on this ambiguity. Under this program, planned before the
War but brought into full operation by a decree of 1 September 1939, some 275,000 people were gassed in centers which
were to be a model for those in which Jews were later exter-
minated. Anyone in a state institution could be sent to the
gas chambers if it was considered that he could not be "re-
habilitated" for useful work. As Dr. Leo Alexander reports,
relying on the testimony of a neuropathologist who received
500 brains from one of the killing centers,

In Germany the exterminations included the mentally de-
fective, psychotics (particularly schizophrenics), epi-
leptics and patients suffering from infirmities of old

Philippa Foot, "Euthanasia," *Philosophy & Public Affairs* 6, no. 2 (Winter 1977). Copyright © 1977 by Philippa
Foot. Reprinted by permission of the author and Princeton University Press.

age and from various organic neurological disorders such
as infantile paralysis, Parkinsonism, multiple sclerosis
and brain tumors...In truth, all those unable to work
and considered nonrehabilitable were killed. (1)

These people were killed because they were "useless" and "a
burden on society"; only the manner of their deaths could be
thought of as relatively easy and quiet.

Let us insist, then, that when we talk about euthanasia
we are talking about a death understood as a good or happy
event for the one who dies. This stipulation follows ety-
mology, but is itself not exactly in line with current usage,
which would be captured by the condition that the death
should not be an evil rather than that it should be a good.
That this is how people talk is shown by the fact that the
case of Karen Ann Quinlan and others in a state of permanent
coma is often discussed under the heading of "euthanasia."
Perhaps it is not too late to object to the use of the word
"euthanasia" in this sense. Apart from the break with the
Greek origins of the word there are other unfortunate aspects
of this extension of the term. For if we say that the death
must be supposed to be a good to the subject we can also
specify that it shall be for his sake that an act of euthanasia is performed. If we say merely that death shall not be
an evil to him, we cannot stipulate that benefiting him shall
be the motive where euthanasia is in question. Given the importance of the question, for whose sake are we acting? it
is good to have a definition of euthanasia which brings under this heading only cases of opting for death for the sake
of the one who dies. Perhaps what is most important is to
say either that euthanasia is to be for the good of the subject or at least that death is to be no evil to him, thus refusing to talk Hitler's language. However, in this paper it
is the first condition that will be understood, with the additional proviso that by an act of euthanasia we mean one of
inducing or otherwise opting for death for the sake of the
one who is to die.

A few lesser points need to be cleared up. In the first
place it must be said that the word "act" is not to be taken
to exclude omission: we shall speak of an act of euthanasia
when someone is deliberately allowed to die, for his own
good, and not only when positive measures are taken to see
that he does. The very general idea we want is that of a
choice of action or inaction directed at another man's death
and causally effective in the sense that, in conjunction
with actual circumstances, it is a sufficient condition of
death. Of complications such as overdetermination, it will
not be necessary to speak.

A second, and definitely minor, point about the definition of an act of euthanasia concerns the question of fact
versus belief. It has already been implied that one who per-
forms an act of euthanasia thinks that death will be merciful
for the subject since we have said that it is on account of
this thought that the act is done. But is it enough that he
acts with this thought, or must things actually be as he
thinks them to be? If one man kills another, or allows him
to die, thinking that he is in the last stages of a terrible
disease, though in fact he could have been cured, is this an
act of euthanasia or not? Nothing much seems to hang on our
decision about this. The same condition has got to enter
into the definition whether as an element in reality or only
as an element in the agent's belief. And however we define
an act of euthanasia culpability or justifiability will be
the same: if a man acts through ignorance his ignorance may
be culpable or it may not. (2)

These are relatively easy problems to solve, but one
that is dauntingly difficult has been passed over in this
discussion of the definition, and must now be faced. It is
easy to say, as if this raised no problems, that an act of
euthanasia is by definition one aiming at the good of the
one whose death is in question, and that it is for his sake
that his death is desired. But how is this to be explained?
Presumably we are thinking of some evil already with him or
to come on him if he continues to live, and death is thought
of as a release from this evil. But this cannot be enough.
Most people's lives contain evils such as grief or pain, but
we do not therefore think that death would be a blessing to
them. On the contrary life is generally supposed to be a
good even for someone who is unusually unhappy or frustrated.
How is it that one can ever wish for death for the sake of
the one who is to die? This difficult question is central to
the discussion of euthanasia, and we shall literally not
know what we are talking about if we ask whether acts of
euthanasia defined as we have defined them are ever morally
permissible without first understanding better the reason
for saying that life is a good, and the possibility that it
is not always so.

If a man should save my life he would be my benefactor.
In normal circumstances this is plainly true; but does one
always benefit another in saving his life? It seems certain
that he does not. Suppose, for instance, that a man were
being tortured to death and was given a drug that lengthened
his sufferings; this would not be a benefit but the reverse.
Or suppose that in a ghetto in Nazi Germany a doctor saved
the life of someone threatened by disease, but that the man
once cured was transported to an extermination camp; the

doctor might wish for the sake of the patient that he had
died of the disease. Nor would a longer stretch of life
always be a benefit to the person who was given it. Compar-
ing Hitler's camps with those of Stalin, Dmitri Panin ob-
serves that in the latter the method of extermination was
made worse by agonies that could stretch out over months.

> Death from a bullet would have been bliss compared
> with what many millions had to endure while dying
> of hunger. The kind of death to which they were
> condemned has nothing to equal it in treachery and
> sadism. (3)

These examples show that to save or prolong a man's life
is not always to do him a service: it may be better for him
if he dies earlier rather than later. It must therefore be
agreed that while life is normally a benefit to the one who
has it, this is not always so.

The judgment is often fairly easy to make--that life is
or is not a good to someone--but the basis for it is very
hard to find. When life is said to be a benefit or a good,
on what grounds is the assertion made?

The difficulty is underestimated if it is supposed that
the problem arises from the fact that one who is dead has
nothing, so that the good someone gets from being alive cannot be compared with the amount he would otherwise have had.
For why should this particular comparison be necessary?
Surely it would be enough if one could say whether or not
someone whose life was prolonged had more good than evil in
the extra stretch of time. Such estimates are not always
possible, but frequently they are; we say, for example, "He
was very happy in those last years," or, "He had little but
unhappiness then." If the balance of good and evil determined whether life was a good to someone we would expect to
find a correlation in the judgments. In fact, of course, we
find nothing of the kind. First, a man who has no doubt
that existence is a good to him may have no idea about the
balance of happiness and unhappiness in his life, or of any
other positive and negative factors that may be suggested.
So the supposed criteria are not always operating where the
judgment is made. And secondly the application of the criteria gives an answer that is often wrong. Many people have
more evil than good in their lives; we do not, however, conclude that we would do these people no service by rescuing
them from death.

To get around this last difficulty Thomas Nagel has
suggested that experience itself is a good which must be

brought in to balance accounts.

> ....life is worth living even when the bad elements
> of experience are plentiful, and the good ones too
> meager to outweigh the bad ones on their own. The
> additional positive weight is supplied by exper-
> ience itself, rather than by any of its contents.

This seems implausible because if experience itself is
a good it must be so even when what we experience is wholly
bad, as in being tortured to death. How should one decide
how much to count for this experiencing; and why count anything at all?

Others have tried to solve the problem by arguing that it
is a man's desire for life that makes us call life a good: if
he wants to live then anyone who prolongs his life does him a
benefit. Yet someone may cling to life where we would say
confidently that it would be better for him if he died, and he
may admit it too. Speaking of those same conditions in which,
as he said, a bullet would have been merciful, Panin writes,

> I should like to pass on my observations concerning
> the absence of suicides under the extremely severe
> conditions of our concentration camps. The more
> that life became desperate, the more a prisoner
> seemed determined to hold onto it. (5)

One might try to explain this by saying that hope was
the ground of this wish to survive for further days and
months in the camp. But there is nothing unintelligible in
the idea that a man might cling to life though he knew those
facts about his future which would make any charitable man
wish that he might die.

The problem remains, and it is hard to know where to
look for a solution. Is there a conceptual connection between life and good? Because life is not always a good we
are apt to reject this idea, and to think that it must be a
contingent fact that life is usually a good, as it is a contingent matter that legacies are usually a benefit, if they
are. Yet it seems not to be a contingent matter that to save
someone's life is ordinarily to benefit him. The problem is
to find where the conceptual connection lies.

It may be good tactics to forget for a time that it is
euthanasia we are discussing and to see how life and good are
connected in the case of living beings other than men. Even
plants have things done to them that are harmful or beneficial, and what does them good must be related in some way to

their living and dying. Let us therefore consider plants
and animals, and then come back to human beings. At least
we shall get away from the temptation to think that the connection between life and benefit must everywhere be a matter
of happiness and unhappiness or of pleasure and pain; the
idea being absurd in the case of animals and impossible even
to formulate for plants.

In case anyone thinks that the concept of the beneficial
applies only in a secondary or analogical way to plants, he
should be reminded that we speak quite straightforwardly in
saying, for instance, that a certain amount of sunlight is
beneficial to most plants. What is in question here is the
habitat in which plants of particular species flourish, but
we can also talk, in a slightly different way, of what does
them good, where there is some suggestion of improvement or
remedy. What has the beneficial to do with sustaining life?
It is tempting to answer, "everything," thinking that a
healthy condition just is the one apt to secure survival. In
fact, however, what is beneficial to a plant may have to do
with reproduction rather than the survival of the individual
member of the species. Nevertheless there is a plain connection between the beneficial and the life-sustaining even for
the individual plant; if something makes it better able to
survive in conditions normal for that species it is <u>ipso
facto</u> good for it. We need go no further, in explaining why
a certain environment or treatment is good for a plant than
to show how it helps this plant to survive. (<u>6</u>)

This connection between the life-sustaining and the
beneficial is reasonably unproblematic, and there is nothing
fanciful or zoomorphic in speaking of benefiting or doing
good to plants. A connection with its survival can make
something beneficial to a plant. But this is not, of course,
to say that we count life as a good to a plant. We may
save its life by giving it what is beneficial; we do not
benefit it by saving its life.

A more ramified concept of benefit is used in speaking
of animal life. New things can be said, such as that an animal is better or worse off for something that happened, or
that it was a good or bad thing for it that it did happen.
And new things count as benefit. In the first place, there
is comfort, which often is, but need not be, related to
health. When loosening a collar which is too tight for a
dog we can say, "That will be better for it." So we see
that the words "better for it" have two different meanings
which we mark when necessary by a difference of emphasis,
saying "better <u>for</u> it" when health is involved. And secondly an animal can be benefited by having its life saved.

"Could you do anything for it?" can be answered by, "Yes, I managed to save its life." Sometimes we may understand this, just as we would for a plant, to mean that we had checked some disease. But we can also do something for an animal by scaring away its predator. If we do this, it is a good thing for the animal that we did, unless of course it immediately meets a more unpleasant end by some other means. Similarly, on the bad side, an animal may be worse off for our intervention, and this not because it pines or suffers but simply because it gets killed.

The problem that vexes us when we think about euthanasia comes on the scene at this point. For if we can do something for an animal--can benefit it--by relieving its suffering but also by saving its life, where does the greater benefit come when only death will end pain? It seemed that life was a good in its own right; yet pain seemed to be an evil with equal status and could therefore make life not a good after all. Is it only life without pain that is a good when animals are concerned? This does not seem a crazy suggestion when we are thinking of animals, since unlike human beings they do not have suffering as part of their normal life. But it is perhaps the idea of ordinary life that matters here. We would not say that we had done anything for an animal if we had merely kept it alive, either in an unconscious state or in a condition where, though conscious, it was unable to operate in an ordinary way; and the fact is that animals in severe and continuous pain simply do not operate normally. So we do not, on the whole, have the option of doing the animal good by saving its life though the life would be a life of pain. No doubt there are borderline cases, but that is no problem. We are not trying to make new judgments possible, but rather to find the principle of the ones we do make.

When we reach human life the problems seem even more troublesome. For now we must take quite new things into account, such as the subject's own view of his life. It is arguable that this places extra constraints on the solution: might it not be counted as a necessary condition of life's being a good to a man that he should see it as such? Is there not some difficulty about the idea that a benefit might be done to him by the saving or prolonging of his life even though he himself wished for death? Of course he might have a quite mistaken view of his own prospects, but let us ignore this and think only of cases where it is life as he knows it that is in question. Can we think that the prolonging of this life would be a benefit to him even though he would rather have it end than continue? (7) It seems that this cannot be ruled out. That there is no simple

incompatibility between life as a good and the wish for death
is shown by the possibility that a man should wish himself
dead, not for his own sake, but for the sake of someone else.
And if we try to amend the thesis to say that life cannot be
a good to one who wishes <u>for his own sake</u> that he should die,
we find the crucial concept slipping through our fingers. As
Bishop Butler pointed out long ago not all ends are either be-
nevolent or self-interested. Does a man wish for death for
his own sake in the relevant sense if, for instance, he
wishes to revenge himself on another by his death. Or what
if he is proud and refuses to stomach dependence or incapacity even though there are many good things left in life for
him? The truth seems to be that the wish for death is sometimes compatible with life's being a good and sometimes not,
which is possible because the description "wishing for death"
is one covering diverse states of mind from that of the determined suicide, pathologically depressed, to that of one who
is surprised to find that the thought of a fatal accident is
viewed with relief. On the one hand, a man may see his life
as a burden but go about his business in a more or less ordinary way; on the other hand, the wish for death may take the
form of a rejection of everything that is in life, as it does
in severe depression. It seems reasonable to say that life
is not a good to one permanently in the latter state, and we
must return to this topic later on.

When are we to say that life is a good or a benefit to a
man? The dilemma that faces us is this. If we say that life
as such is a good we find ourselves refuted by the examples
given at the beginning of this discussion. We therefore in-
clide to think that it is as bringing good things that life
is a good, where it is a good. But if life is a good only
because it is the condition of good things, why is it not
equally an evil when it brings bad things? And how can it be
a good even when it brings more evil than good?

It should be noted that the problem has here been form-
ulated in terms of the balance of good and evil, not that of
happiness and unhappiness, and that it is not to be solved by
the denial (which may be reasonable enough) that unhappiness
is the only evil or happiness the only good. In this paper
no view has been expressed about the nature of goods other
than life itself. The point is that on any view of the goods
and evils that life can contain, it seems that a life with
more evil than good could still itself be a good.

It may be useful to review the judgments with which our
theory must square. Do we think that life can be a good to
one who suffers a lot of pain? Clearly we do. What about
severely handicapped people; can life be a good to them?

Clearly it can be, for even if someone is almost completely
paralyzed, perhaps living in an iron lung, perhaps able to
move things only by means of a tube held between his lips, we
do not rule him out of order if he says that some benefactor
saved his life. Nor is it different with mental handicap.
There are many fairly severely handicapped people--such as
those with Down's Syndrome (Mongolism)--for whom a simple affectionate life is possible. What about senility? Does this
break the normal connection between life and good? Here we
must surely distinguish between forms of senility. Some
forms leave a life which we count someone as better off having than not having, so that a doctor who prolonged it would
benefit the person concerned. With some kinds of senility
this is however no longer true. There are some in geriatric
wards who are barely conscious, though they can move a little
and swallow food put into their mouths. To prolong such a
state, whether in the old or in the very severely mentally
handicapped is not to do them a service or confer a benefit.
But of course it need not be the reverse: only if there is
suffering would one wish for the sake of the patient that
he should die.

It seems, therefore, that merely being alive even without suffering is not a good, and that we must make a distinction similar to that which we made when animals were our topic. But how is the line to be drawn in the case of men?
What is to count as ordinary human life in the relevant sense?
If it were only the very senile or very ill who were to be
said not to have this life it might seem right to describe it
in terms of operation. But it will be hard to find the sense
in which the men described by Panin were not operating, given
that they dragged themselves out to the forest to work. What
is it about the life that the prisoners were living that
makes us put it on the other side of the dividing line from
that of some severely ill or suffering patients, and from
most of the physically or mentally handicapped? It is not
that they were in captivity, for life in captivity can certainly be a good. Nor is it merely the unusual nature of
their life. In some ways the prisoners were living more as
other men do than the patient in an iron lung.

The suggested solution to the problem is, then, that
there is a certain conceptual connection between life and
good in the case of human beings as in that of animals and
even plants. Here, as there, however, it is not the mere
state of being alive that can determine, or itself count as,
a good, but rather life coming up to some standard of normal-
ity. It was argued that it is as part of ordinary life that
the elements of good that a man may have are relevant to the
question of whether saving his life counts as benefiting him.

Ordinary human lives, even very hard lives, contain a minimum of basic goods, but when these are absent the idea of
life is no longer linked to that of good. And since it is in
this way that the elements of good contained in a man's life
are relevant to the question of whether he is benefited if
his life is preserved, there is no reason why it should be
the balance of good and evil that counts.

It should be added that evils are relevant in one way
when, as in the examples discussed above, they destroy the
possibility of ordinary goods, but in a different way when
they invade a life from which the goods are already absent
for a different reason. So, for instance, the connection between life and good may be broken because consciousness has
sunk to a very low level, as in extreme senility or severe
brain damage. In itself this kind of life seems to be
neither good nor evil, but if suffering sets in one would
hope for a speedy end.

The idea we need seems to be that of life which is ordinary human life in the following respect--that it contains a
minimum of basic human goods. What is ordinary in human
life--even in very hard lives--is that a man is not driven to
work far beyond his capacity; that he has the support of a
family or community; that he can more or less satisfy his
hunger; that he has hopes for the future; that he can lie
down to rest at night. Such things were denied to the men in
the Vyatlag camps described by Panin; not even rest at night
was allowed them when they were tormented by bed-bugs, by
noise and stench, and by routines such as body-searches and
bath-parades--arranged for the night time so that work norms
would not be reduced. Disease too can so take over a man's
life that the normal human goods disappear. When a patient
is so overwhelmed by pain or nausea that he cannot eat with
pleasure, if he can eat at all, and is out of the reach of
even the most loving voice, he no longer has ordinary human
life in the sense in which the words are used here. And we
may now pick up a thread from an earlier part of the discussion by remarking that crippling depression can destroy the
enjoyment of ordinary goods as effectively as external circumstances can remove them.

This, admittedly inadequate, discussion of the sense in
which life is normally a good, and of the reasons why it may
not be so in some particular case, completes the account of
what euthanasia is here taken to be. An act of euthanasia,
whether literally act or rather omission, is attributed to an
agent who opts for the death of another because in his case
life seems to be an evil rather than a good. The question
now to be asked is whether acts of euthanasia are ever

justifiable. But there are two topics here rather than one.
For it is one thing to say that some acts of euthanasia considered only in themselves and their results are morally un-
objectionable, and another to say that it would be all right
to legalize them. Perhaps the practice of euthanasia would
allow too many abuses, and perhaps there would be too many
mistakes. Moreover the practice might have very important
and highly undesirable side effects, because it is unlikely
that we could change our principles about the treatment of
the old and the ill without changing fundamental emotional attitudes and social relations. The topics must, therefore, be
treated separately. In the next part of the discussion, nothing will be said about the social consequences and possible
abuses of the practice of euthanasia, but only about acts of
euthanasia considered in themselves.

What we want to know is whether acts of euthanasia, defined as we have defined them, are ever morally permissible.
To be more accurate, we want to know whether it is ever sufficient justification of the choice of death for another that
death can be counted a benefit rather than harm, and that
this is why the choice is made.

It will be impossible to get a clear view of the area to
which this topic belongs without first marking the distinct
grounds on which objection may lie when one man opts for the
death of another. There are two different virtues whose requirements are, in general, contrary to such actions. An un-
justified act of killing, or allowing to die, is contrary to
justice or to charity, or to both virtues, and the moral
failings are distinct. Justice has to do with what men owe
each other in the way of noninterference and positive service.
When used in this wide sense, which has its history in the
doctrine of the cardinal virtues, justice is not especially
connected with, for instance, law courts but with the whole
area of rights, and duties corresponding to rights. Thus
murder is one form of injustice, dishonesty another, and
wrongful failure to keep contracts a third; chicanery in a
law court or defrauding someone of his inheritance are simply
other cases of injustice. Justice as such is not directly
linked to the good of another, and may require that something
be rendered to him even where it will do him harm, as Hume
pointed out when he remarked that a debt must be paid even to
a profligate debauchee who "would rather receive harm than
benefit from large possessions." (7) Charity, on the other
hand, is the virtue which attaches us to the good of others.
An act of charity is in question only where something is not
demanded by justice, but a lack of charity and of justice can
be shown where a man is denied something which he both needs
and has a right to; both charity and justice demand that

widows and orphans are not defrauded, and the man who cheats them is neither charitable nor just.

It is easy to see that the two grounds of objection to inducing death are distinct. A murder is an act of injustice. A culpable failure to come to the aid of someone whose life is threatened is normally contrary, not to justice, but to charity. But where one man is under contract, explicit or implicit, to come to the aid of another injustice too will be shown. Thus injustice may be involved either in an act or an omission, and the same is true of a lack of charity; charity may demand that someone be aided, but also that an unkind word not be spoken.

The distinction between charity and justice will turn out to be of the first importance when voluntary and non-voluntary euthanasia are distinguished later on. This is because of the connection between justice and rights, and something should now be said about this. I believe it is true to say that wherever a man acts unjustly he has infringed a right, since justice has to do with whatever a man is owed, and whatever he is owed is his as a matter of right. Something should therefore be said about the different kinds of rights. The distinction commonly made is between having a right in the sense of having a liberty, and having a "claim-right" or "right of recipience." (8) The best way to understand such a distinction seems to be as follows. To say that a man has a right in the sense of a liberty is to say that no one can demand that he do not do the thing which he has a right to do. The fact that he has a right to do it consists in the fact that a certain kind of objection does not lie against his doing it. Thus a man has a right in this sense to walk down a public street or park his car in a public parking space. It does not follow that no one else may prevent him from doing so. If for some reason I want a certain man not to park in a certain place I may lawfully park there myself or get my friends to do so, thus preventing him from doing what he has a right (in the sense of a liberty) to do. It is different, however, with a claim-right. This is the kind of right which I have in addition to a liberty when, for example, I have a private parking space; now others have duties in the way of noninterference, as in this case, or of service, as in the case where my claim-right is to goods or services promised to me. Sometimes one of these rights gives other people the duty of securing to me that to which I have a right, but at other times their duty is merely to refrain from interference. If a fall of snow blocks my private parking space there is normally no obligation for anyone else to clear it away. Claim rights generate duties; sometimes these duties are duties of noninterference; sometimes they are

duties of service. If your right gives me the duty not to
interfere with you I have "no right" to do it; similarly, if
your right gives me the duty to provide something for you I
have "no right" to refuse to do it. What I lack is the right
which is a liberty; I am not "at liberty" to interfere with
you or to refuse the service.

Where in this picture does the right to life belong? No
doubt people have the right to live in the sense of a liberty,
but what is important is the cluster of claim-rights brought
together under the title of the right to life. The chief of
these is, of course, the right to be free from interferences
that threaten life. If other people aim their guns at us or
try to pour poison into our drink we can, to put it mildly,
demand that they desist. And then there are the services we
can claim from doctors, health officers, bodyguards, and
firemen; the rights that depend on contract or public arrangement. Perhaps there is no particular point in saying that
the duties these people owe us belong to the right to life;
we might as well say that all the services owed to anyone by
tailors, dressmakers, and couturiers belong to a right called
the right to be elegant. But contracts such as those understood in the patient-doctor relationship come in an important
way when we are discussing the rights and wrongs of euthanasia, and are therefore mentioned here.

Do people have the right to what they need in order to
survive, apart from the right conferred by special contracts
into which other people have entered for the supplying of
these necessities? Do people in the underdeveloped countries
in which starvation is rife have the right to the food they
so evidently lack? Joel Feinberg, discussing this question,
suggests that they should be said to have "a claim," distinguishing this from a "valid claim," which gives a claim-right.

> The manifesto writers on the other side who seem to
> identify needs, or at least basic needs, with what
> they call "human rights," are more properly des-
> cribed, I think, as urging upon the world community
> the moral principle that all basic human needs
> ought to be recognized as claims (in the customary
> prima facie sense) worthy of sympathy and serious
> consideration right now, even though, in many cases,
> they cannot yet plausibly be treated as valid
> claims, that is, as grounds of any other people's
> duties. This way of talking avoids the anomaly of
> ascribing to all human beings now, even those in
> pre-industrial societies, such "economic and social
> rights" as "periodic holidays with pay." (9)

This seems reasonable, though we notice that there are some actual rights to service which are not based on anything like a contract, as for instance the right that children have to support from their parents and parents to support from their children in old age, though both sets of rights are to some extent dependent on existing social arrangements.

Let us now ask how the right to life affects the morality of acts of euthanasia. Are such acts sometimes or always ruled out by the right to life? This is certainly a possibility; for although an act of euthanasia is, by our definition, a matter of opting for death for the good of the one who is to die, there is, as we noted earlier, no direct connection between that to which a man has a right and that which is for his good. It is true that men have the right only to the kind of thing that is, in general, a good: we do not think that people have the right to garbage or polluted air. Nevertheless, a man may have the right to something which he himself would be better off without; where rights exist it is a man's will that counts, not his or anyone else's estimate of benefit or harm. So the duties complementary to the right to life—the general duty of noninterference and the duty of service incurred by certain persons—are not affected by the quality of a man's life or by his prospects. Even if it is true that he would be, as we say, "better off dead," so long as he wants to live, this does not justify us in killing him and may not justify us in deliberately allowing him to die. All of us have the duty of noninterference, and some of us may have the duty to sustain his life. Suppose, for example, that a retreating army has to leave behind wounded or exhausted soldiers in the wastes of an arid or snowbound land where the only prospect is death by starvation or at the hands of an enemy notoriously cruel. It has often been the practice to accord a merciful bullet to men in such desperate straits. But suppose that one of them demands that he should be left alive? It seems clear that his comrades have no right to kill him, though it is a quite different question as to whether they should give him a life-prolonging drug. The right to life can sometimes give a duty of positive service, but does not do so here. What it does give is the right to be left alone.

Interestingly enough we have arrived by way of a consideration of the right to life at the distinction normally labeled "active" versus "passive" euthanasia, and often thought to be irrelevant to the moral issue. (10) Once it is seen that the right to life is a distinct ground of objection to certain acts of euthanasia, and that this right creates a duty of noninterference more widespread than the duties of care there can be no doubt about the relevance of the distinction between passive and active euthanasia. Where everyone may have the duty to leave someone alone, it may be that no one has the duty to maintain his life, or that only some people do.

Where then do the boundaries of the "active" and "passive" lie? In some ways the words are themselves misleading, because they suggest the difference between act and omission which is not quite what we want. Certainly the act of shooting someone is the kind of thing we were talking about under the heading of "interference," and omitting to give him a drug a case of refusing care. But the act of turning off a respirator should surely be thought of as no different from the decision not to start it; if doctors had decided that a patient should be allowed to die, either course of action might follow, and both should be counted as passive rather than active euthanasia if euthanasia were in question. The point seems to be that interference in a course of treatment is not the same as other interference in a man's life, and particularly if the same body of people are responsible for the treatment and for its discontinuance. In such a case we could speak of the disconnecting of the apparatus as killing the man, or of the hospital as allowing him to die. By and large, it is the act of killing that is ruled out under the heading of noninterference, but not in every case.

Doctors commonly recognize this distinction, and the grounds on which some philosophers have denied it seem untenable. James Rachels, for instance, believes that if the difference between active and passive is relevant anywhere, it should be relevant everywhere, and he has pointed to an example in which it seems to make no difference which is done. If someone saw a child drowning in a bath it would seem just as bad to let it drown as to push its head under water. (11) If "it makes no difference" means that one act would be as iniquitous as the other this is true. It is not that killing is worse than allowing to die, but that the two are contrary to distinct virtues, which gives the possibility that in some circumstances one is impermissible and the other permissible. In the circumstances invented by Rachels, both are wicked: it is contrary to justice to push the child's head under the water--something one has no right to do. To leave it to drown is not contrary to justice, but it is a particularly glaring example of lack of charity. Here it makes no practical difference because the requirements of justice and charity coincide; but in the case of the retreating army they did not: charity would have required that the wounded soldier be killed had not justice required that he be left alive. (12) In such a case it makes all the difference whether a man opts for the death of another in a positive action, or whether he allows him to die. An analogy with the right to property will make the point clear. If a man owns something he has the right to it even when its possession does him harm, and we have no right to take it from him. But if one day it should blow away, maybe nothing requires us to get it back for him; we could not deprive him of it, but we may allow it to go. This is not to deny that it will often be an unfriendly act or one based on an arrogant judgment when we refuse to do what he wants. Nevertheless, we would be within our rights, and it might be that no moral objection of any kind would lie against our refusal.

It is important to emphasize that a man's rights may stand between us and the action we would dearly like to take for his sake. They may, of course, also prevent action which we would like to take for the sake of others, as when it might be tempting to kill one man to save several. But it is interesting that the limits of allowable interference, however uncertain, seem stricter in the first case than the second. Perhaps there are no cases in which it would be all right to kill a man against his will <u>for his own sake</u> unless they could equally well be described as cases of allowing him to die, as in the example of turning off the respirator. However, there are circumstances, even if these are very rare, in which one man's life would justifiably be sacrificed to save others, and "killing" would be the only description of what was being done. For instance, a vehicle which had gone out of control might be steered from a path on which it would not be permissible to steer a vehicle towards someone in order to kill him, against his will, for his own good. An analogy with property rights illustrates the point. One may not destroy a man's property against his will on the grounds that he would be better off without it; there are however circumstances in which it could be destroyed for the sake of others, If his house is liable to fall and kill him that is his affair; it might, however, without injustice be destroyed to stop the spread of a fire.

We see then that the distinction between active and passive, important as it is elsewhere, has a special importance in the area of euthanasia. It should also be clear why James Rachels' other argument, that it is often "more humane" to kill than to allow to die, does not show that the distinction between active and passive euthanasia is morally irrelevant. It might be "more humane" in this sense to deprive a man of the property that brings evils on him, or to refuse to pay what is owed to Hume's profligate debauchee; but if we say this we must admit that an act which is "more humane" than its alternative may be morally objectionable because it infringes rights.

So far we have said very little about the right to service as opposed to the right to noninterference, though it was agreed that both might be brought under the heading of "the right to life." What about the duty to preserve life that may belong to special classes of persons such as bodyguards, firemen, or doctors? Unlike the general public they are not within their rights if they merely refrain from interfering and do not try to sustain life. The subject's claim-rights are two-fold as far as they are concerned and passive as well as active euthanasia may be ruled out here if it is against his will. This is not to say that he has the right to any and every service needed to save or prolong his life; the rights of other people set limits to what may be demanded, both because they have the right not to be interfered with and because they may have a competing right to services. Furthermore one must enquire just what the contract or implicit agreement amounts to in each case. Firemen and bodyguards presumably have a duty which is simply to preserve life, within the limits of justice to others and of reasonableness to themselves. With doctors it may however be different, since their duty relates not only to preserving life but also to the relief of suffering. It is not clear what a doctor's duties are to his patient if life can be prolonged only at the cost of suffering or suffering relieved only by measures that shorten life. George Fletcher has argued that what the doctor is under contract to do depends on what is generally done, because this is what a patient will reasonably expect. (14) This seems right. If procedures are part of normal medical practice then it seems that the patient can demand them however much it may be against his interest to do so. Once again it is not a matter of what is "most humane."

That the patient's right to life may set limits to permissible acts of euthanasia seems undeniable. If he does not want to die no one has the right to practice active euthanasia on him, and passive euthanasia may also be ruled out where he has a right to the services of doctors or others.

Perhaps few will deny what has so far been said about the impermissibility of acts of euthanasia simply because we have so far spoken about the case of one who positively wants to live, and about his rights, whereas those who advocate euthanasia are usually thinking either about those who wish to die or about those whose wishes cannot be ascertained either because they cannot properly be said to have wishes or because, for one reason or another, we are unable to form a reliable estimate of what they are. The question that must

now be asked is whether the latter type of case, where euthanasia though not involuntary would again be nonvoluntary, is
different from the one discussed so far. Would we have the
right to kill someone for his own good so long as we had no
idea that he positively wished to live? And what about the
life-prolonging duties of doctors in the same circumstances?
This is a very difficult problem. On the one hand, it seems
ridiculous to suppose that a man's right to life is something
which generates duties only where he has signaled that he
wants to live; as a borrower does indeed have a duty to return something lent on indefinite loan only if the lender in-
dicates that he wants it back. On the other hand, it might
be argued that there is something illogical about the idea
that a right has been infringed if someone incapable of saying whether he wants it or not is deprived of something that
is doing him harm rather than good. Yet on the analogy of
property we would say that a right has been infringed. Only
if someone had earlier told us that in such circumstances he
would not want to keep the thing could we think that his
right had been waived. Perhaps if we could make confident
judgments about what anyone in such circumstances would wish,
or what he would have wished beforehand had he considered the
matter, we could agree to consider the right to life as "dor-
mant," needing to be asserted if the normal duties were to
remain. But as things are we cannot make any such assumption;
we simply do not know what most people would want, or would
have wanted, us to do unless they tell us. This is certainly
the case so far as active measures to end life are concerned.
Possibly it is different, or will become different, in the
matter of being kept alive, so general is the feeling against
using sophisticated procedures on moribund patients, and so
much is this dreaded by people who are old or terminally ill.
Once again the distinction between active and passive euthanasia has come on the scene, but this time because most
people's attitudes to the two are so different. It is just
possible that we might presume, in the absence of specific
evidence, that someone would not wish, beyond a certain
point, to be kept alive; it is certainly not possible to assume that he would wish to be killed.

In the last paragraph we have begun to broach the topic
of voluntary euthanasia, and this we must now discuss. What
is to be said about the case in which there is no doubt
about someone's wish to die: either he has told us beforehand
that he would wish it in circumstances such as he is now in,
and has shown no sign of a change of mind, or else he tells
us now, being in possession of his faculties and of a steady
mind. We should surely say that the objections previously
urged against acts of euthanasia, which it must be remembered
were all on the ground of rights, had disappeared. It does

not seem that one would infringe someone's right to life in
killing him with his permission and in fact at his request.
Why should someone not be able to waive his right to life, or
rather, as would be more likely to happen, to cancel some of
the duties of noninterference that this right entails? (He
is more likely to say that he should be killed by this man at
this time in this manner, than to say that anyone may kill
him at any time and in any way.) Similarly someone may give
permission for the destruction of his property, and request
it. The important thing is that he gives a critical permission, and it seems that this is enough to cancel the duty
normally associated with the right. If someone gives you
permission to destroy it can no longer be said that you have
no right to do so, and I do not see why it should not be the
case with taking a man's life. An objection might be made on
the ground that only God has the right to take life, but in
this paper religious as opposed to moral arguments are being
left aside. Religion apart, there seems to be no case to be
made out for an infringement of rights if a man who wishes to
die is allowed to die or even killed. But of course it does
not follow that there is no moral objection to it. Even with
property, which is after all a relatively small matter, one
might be wrong to destroy what one had the right to destroy.
For, apart from its value to other people, it might be valuable to the man who wanted it destroyed, and charity might
require us to hold our hand where justice did not.

Let us review the conclusion of this part of the argument, which has been about euthanasia and the right to life.
It has been argued that from this side come stringent restrictions on the acts of euthanasia that could be morally
permissible. Active nonvoluntary euthanasia is ruled out by
that part of the right to life which creates the duty of noninterference though passive nonvoluntary euthanasia is not
ruled out, except where the right to life-preserving action
has been created by some special condition such as a contract
between a man and his doctor, and it is not always certain
just what such a contract involves. Voluntary euthanasia is
another matter: as the preceding paragraph suggested, no
right is infringed if a man is allowed to die or even killed
at his own request.

Turning now to the other objection that normally holds
against inducing the death of another, that it is against
charity, or benevolence, we must tell a very different story.
Charity is the virtue that gives attachment to the good of
others, and because life is normally a good, charity normally
demands that it should be saved or prolonged. But as we so
defined an act of euthanasia that it seeks a man's death for
his own sake--for his good--charity will normally speak in

favor of it. This is not, of course, to say that charity can
require an act of contrary to justice--that is, it does not
infringe rights--charity will rather be in its favor than
against.

Once more the distinction between nonvoluntary and voluntary euthanasia must be considered. Could it ever be compatible with charity to seek a man's death although he wanted
to live, or at least had not let us know that he wanted to
die? It has been argued that in such circumstances active
euthanasia would infringe his right to life, but passive
euthanasia would not do so, unless he had some special right
to life-preserving service from the one who allowed him to
die. What would charity dictate? Obviously when a man wants
to live there is a presumption that he will be benefited if
his life is prolonged, and if it is so the question of euthanasia does not arise. But it is, on the other hand, possible that he wants to live where it would be better for him
to die: perhaps he does not realize the desperate situation
he is in, or perhaps he is afraid of dying. So, in spite of
a very proper resistance to refusing to go along with a man's
own wishes in the matter of life and death, someone might
justifiably refuse to prolong the life even of someone who
asked him to prolong it, as in the case of refusing to give
the wounded soldier a drug that would keep him alive to meet
a terrible end. And it is even more obvious that charity
does not always dictate that life should be prolonged where a
man's own wishes, hypothetical or actual, are not known.

So much for the relation of charity to nonvoluntary passive euthanasia, which was not, like nonvoluntary active
euthanasia, ruled out by the right to life. Let us now ask
what charity has to say about voluntary euthanasia both active and passive. It was suggested in the discussion of justice that if of sound mind and steady desire a man might give
others the right to allow him to die or even to kill him,
where otherwise this would be ruled out. But it was pointed
out that this would not settle the question of whether the
act was morally permissible, and it is this that we must now
consider. Could not charity speak against what justice allowed? Indeed it might do so. For while the fact that a man
wants to die suggests that his life is wretched, and while
his rejection of life may itself tend to take the good out
of the things he might have enjoyed, nevertheless his wish to
die might here be opposed for his own sake just as it might
be if suicide were in question. Perhaps there is hope that
his mental condition will improve. Perhaps he is mistaken
in thinking his disease incurable. Perhaps he wants to die
for the sake of someone else on whom he feels he is a burden,
and we are not ready to accept this sacrifice whether for

ourselves or others. In such cases, and there will surely be
many of them, it could not be for his own sake that we kill
him or allow him to die, and therefore euthanasia as defined
in this paper would not be in question. But this is not to
deny that there could be acts of voluntary euthanasia both
passive and active against which neither justice nor charity
would speak.

We have now considered the morality of euthanasia both
voluntary and nonvoluntary, and active and passive. The conclusion has been that nonvoluntary active euthanasia (roughly,
killing a man against his will or without his consent) is
never justified; that is to say, that a man's being killed
for his own good never justifies the act unless he himself
has consented to it. A man's rights are infringed by such an
action, and it is therefore contrary to justice. However,
all the other combinations, nonvoluntary passive euthanasia,
voluntary active euthanasia, and voluntary passive euthanasia
are sometimes compatible with both justice and charity. But
the strong condition carried in the definition of euthanasia
adopted in this paper must not be forgotten; an act of euthanasia as here understood is one whose purpose is to benefit
the one who dies.

In the light of this discussion let us look at our present practices. Are they good or are they bad? And what
changes might be made, thinking now not only of the morality
of particular acts of euthanasia but also of the indirect
effects of instituting different practices of the abuses to
which they might be subject and of the changes that might
come about if euthanasia became a recognized part of the
social scene.

The first thing to notice is that it is wrong to ask
whether we should introduce the practice of euthanasia as if
it were not something we already had. In fact we do have it.
For instance it is common, where the medical prognosis is
very bad, for doctors to recommend against measures to prolong life, and particularly where a process of degeneration
producing one medical emergency after another has already set
in. If these doctors are not certainly within their legal
rights this is something that is apt to come as a surprise to
them as to the general public. It is also obvious that euthanasia is often practiced where old people are concerned. If
someone very old and soon to die is attacked by a disease
that makes his life wretched, doctors do not always come in
with life-prolonging drugs. Perhaps poor patients are more
fortunate in this respect than rich patients, being more
often left to die in peace; but it is in any case a well recognized piece of medical practice, which is a form of euth-

anasia.

'   No doubt the case of infants with mental or physical defects will be suggested as another example of the practice of
euthanasia as we already have it, since such infants are
sometimes deliberately allowed to die. That they are deliberately allowed to die is certain; children with severe spina
bifida malformations are not always operated on even when it
is thought that without the operation they will die; and even
in the case of children with Down's Syndrome who have intestinal obstructions the relatively simple operation that would
make it possible to feed them is sometimes not performed. (15)
Whether this is euthanasia in our sense or only as the Nazis
understood it is another matter. We must ask the crucial
question, "Is it for the sake of the child himself that the
doctors and parents choose his death?" In some cases the
answer may really be yes, and what is more important, it may
really be true that the kind of life which is a good is not
possible or likely for this child, and that there is little
but suffering and frustration in store for him. (16)   But
this must presuppose that the medical prognosis is wretchedly
bad, as it may be for some spina bifida children. With children who are born with Down's Syndrome it is, however, quite
different. Most of these are able to live on for quite a
time in a reasonably contented way, remaining like children
all their lives but capable of affectionate relationships and
able to play games and perform simple tasks. The fact is, of
course, that the doctors who recommend against life-saving
procedures for handicapped infants are usually thinking not
of them but rather of their parents and of other children in
the family or of the "burden on society" if the children survive. So it is not for their sake but to avoid trouble to
others that they are allowed to die. When brought out into
the open this seems unacceptable: at least we do not easily
accept the principle that adults who need special care should
be counted too burdensome to be kept alive. It must in any
case be insisted that if children with Down's Syndrome are
deliberately allowed to die this is not a matter of euthanasia except in Hitler's sense. And for our children, since
we scruple to gas them, not even the manner of their death is
"quiet and easy"; when not treated for an intestinal obstruc-
tion a baby simply starves to death. Perhaps some will take
this as an argument for allowing active euthanasia, in which
case they will be in the company of an S.S. man stationed in
the Warthgenau who sent Eichmann a memorandum telling him
that "Jews in the coming winter could no longer be fed" and
submitting for his consideration a proposal as to whether "it
would not be the most humane solution to kill those Jews who
were incapable of work through some quicker means." (17)   If
we say we are unable to look after children with handicaps we

are no more telling the truth than was the S.S. man who said
that the Jews could not be fed.

Nevertheless if it is ever right to allow deformed children to die because life will be a misery to them, or not to
take measures to prolong for a little the life of a newborn
baby whose life cannot extend beyond a few months of intense
medical intervention, there is a genuine problem about active
as opposed to passive euthanasia. There are well-known cases
in which the medical staff has looked on wretchedly while an
infant died slowly from starvation and dehydration because
they did not feel able to give a lethal injection. According
to the principles discussed in the earlier part of this paper
they would indeed have had no right to give it, since an infant cannot ask that it should be done. The only possible
solution--supposing that voluntary active euthanasia were to
be legalized--would be to appoint guardians to act on the infant's behalf. In a different climate of opinion this might
not be dangerous, but at present, when people so readily assume that the life of a handicapped baby is of no value, one
would be loath to support it.

Finally, on the subject of handicapped children, another
word should be said about those with severe mental defects.
For them too it might sometimes be right to say that one
would wish for death for their sake. But not even severe
mental handicap automatically brings a child within the scope
even of a possible act of euthanasia. If the level of consciousness is low enough it could not be said that life is a
good to them, any more than in the case of those suffering
from extreme senility. Nevertheless if they do not suffer it
will not be an act of euthanasia by which someone opts for
their death. Perhaps charity does not demand that strenuous
measures are taken to keep people in this state alive, but
euthanasia does not come into the matter, any more than it
does when someone is, like Karen Ann Quinlan, in a state of
permanent coma. Much could be said about this last case. It
might even be suggested that in the case of unconsciousness
this "life" is not the life to which "the right to life" re-
fers. But that is not our topic here.

What we must consider, even if only briefly, is the possibility that euthanasia, genuine euthanasia, and not contrary to the requirements of justice or charity, should be
legalized over a wider area. Here we are up against the
really serious problem of abuse. Many people want, and want
very badly, to be rid of their elderly relatives and even of
their ailing husbands or wives. Would any safeguards ever be
able to stop them describing as euthanasia what was really
for their own benefit? And would it be possible to prevent

the occurrence of acts which were genuinely acts of euthanasia but morally impermissible because infringing the rights of a patient who wished to live?

Perhaps the furthest we should go is to encourage patients to make their own contracts with a doctor by making it known whether they wish him to prolong their life in case of painful terminal illness or of incapacity. A document such as the Living Will seems eminently sensible, and should surely be allowed to give a doctor following the previously expressed wishes of the patient immunity from legal proceedings by relatives. (18) Legalizing active euthanasia is, however, another matter. Apart from the special repugnance doctors feel towards the idea of a lethal injection, it may be of the very greatest importance to keep a psychological barrier up against killing. Moreover it is active euthanasia which is the most liable to abuse. Hitler would not have been able to kill 275,000 people in his "euthanasia" program if he had had to wait for them to need life-saving treatment. But there are other objections to active euthanasia, even voluntary active euthanasia. In the first place it would be hard to devise procedures that would protect people from being persuaded into giving their consent. And secondly the possibility of active voluntary euthanasia might change the social scene in ways that would be very bad. As things are, people do, by and large, expect to be looked after if they are old or ill. This is one of the good things that we have, but we might lose it, and be much worse off without it. It might come to be expected that someone likely to need a lot of looking after should call for the doctor and demand his own death. Something comparable could be good in an extremely poverty-stricken community where the children genuinely suffered from lack of food; but in rich societies such as ours it would surely be a spiritual disaster. Such possibilities should make us very wary of supporting large measures of euthanasia, even where moral principle applied to the individual act does not rule it out.

Footnotes

I would like to thank Derek Parfit and the editors of
Philosophy & Public Affairs (in which this essay made its
first appearance) for their very helpful comments.

1. Leo Alexander, "Medical Science under Dictatorship," New
   England Journal of Medicine, 14 July 1949, p. 40.

2. For a discussion of culpable and nonculpable ignorance
   see Thomas Aquinas, Summa Theologica, First Part of the
   Second Part, Question 6, article 8, and Question 19, articles 5 and 6.

3. Dmitri Panin, The Notebooks of Sologdin (London, 1976),
   pp. 66-67.

4. Thomas Nagel, "Death," in James Rachels, ed., Moral Problems (New York, 1971), p. 362.

5. Panin, Sologdin, p. 85.

6. Yet some detail needs to be filled in to explain why we
   should not say that a scarecrow is beneficial to plants
   it protects. Perhaps what is beneficial must either be
   a feature of the plant itself, such as protective
   prickles, or else must work on the plant directly, such
   as a line of trees which give it shade.

7. David Hume, Treatise, Book III, Part II, Section I.

8. See, for example D.D. Raphael, "Human Rights Old and
   New," in D.D. Raphael, ed., Political Theory and the
   Rights of Man (London, 1967), and Joel Feinberg, "The
   Nature and Value of Rights," The Journal of Value Inquiry
   4, no. 4 (Winter 1970): 243-257. Reprinted in Samuel
   Gorovitz, ed., Moral Problems in Medicine (Englewood
   Cliffs, New Jersey, 1976).

9. Feinberg, "Human Rights," Moral Problems in Medicine,
   p. 465.

10. See, for example, James Rachels, "Active and Passive
    Euthanasia," New England Journal of Medicine 292, no. 2
    (9 Jan. 1975): 78-80.

11. Ibid.

12. It is not, however, that justice and charity conflict. A

man does not lack charity because he refrains from an
act of injustice which would have been for someone's
good.

13. For a discussion of such questions, see my article "The
    Problem of Abortion and the Doctrine of Double Effect,"
    Oxford Review, no. 5 (1967): reprinted in Rachels,
    Moral Problems, and Gorovitz, Moral Problems in Medicine.

14. George Fletcher "Legal Aspects of the Decision not to
    Prolong Life," Journal of the American Medical Associa-
    tion 203, no. 1 (1 Jan. 1968): 119-122. Reprinted in
    Gorovitz.

15. I have been told this by a pediatrician in a well-known
    medical center in the United States. It is confirmed
    by Anthony M. Shaw and Iris A. Shaw, "Dilemma of In-
    formed Consent in Children," The New England Journal of
    Medicine 289, no. 17 (25 Oct. 1973): 885-890. Reprinted
    in Gorovitz.

16. It must be remembered, however, that many of the social
    miseries of spina bifida children could be avoided.
    Professor R.B. Zachary is surely right to insist on
    this. See, for example, "Ethical and Social Aspects of
    Spina Bifida," The Lancet, 3 Aug. 1968, pp. 274-276.
    Reprinted in Gorovitz.

17. Quoted by Hannah Arendt, Eichmann in Jerusalem (London
    1963), p. 90.

18. Details of this document are to be found in J.A. Behnke
    and Sissela Bok, eds., The Dilemmas of Euthanasia (New
    York, 1975), and in A.B. Downing, ed., Euthanasia and
    the Right to Life: The Case for Voluntary Euthanasia
    (London, 1969).

The Right to Die and the Obligation to Care: Allowing to Die, Killing for Mercy, and Suicide

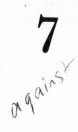

William F. May

When we assert human rights, we usually do so with some awareness of social, cultural, and political forces that would deny them. Thus our own bill of rights -- including freedom of speech, assembly, and worship, and the right to bear arms -- sprang from a healthy suspicion of those institutions -- political and ecclesiastical -- that threatened to deprive a citizenry of its due. When people, therefore, get concerned about the right to die, against what forces are they girding themselves when they assert the right?

In the view of some critics, the major cultural and social force opposed to the right to die is the ancient and continuing philosophical and theological tradition of the West. Commentators reach this conclusion citing the classical Christian opposition to suicide. For natural law theorists among the Christians, suicide was not only immoral but profoundly <u>unnatural</u> -- literally, suicide violates our nature. One of the laws of nature, so the argument goes, is the law of self-preservation. This law is the first principle of nature within us and the precondition of all else. No one has the natural right to kill himself or to expect others to assist him in so doing.

Since God is the source and ground for the laws of nature, theologians called suicide not only immoral and unnatural, but sinful: a breach of divine command. Accomplices were thus guilty of the sin of murder. Successful suicides were not granted traditional funeral rites, i.e., Christian burial. Worse, popular reaction led to the abuse of the suicide's corpse and the persecution and humiliation of the unsuccessful suicide. The theologian defined suicide as sin and the population at large was disposed to punish the sinner.

The weight of the legal tradition of the West has similarly opposed the right to die. Self-destruction was not
only immoral, unnatural, and sinful, but illegal. Suicide,
to be sure, was a rather special crime; the successful per-
petrator was able to remove himself permanently from the
reach of social punishment. But only to a degree. The suicide knew beforehand, after all, that his family might be
humiliated and his body degraded. Once again, any who
assisted in this peculiar crime were considered murderers.

While the cumulative philosophical, theological, and
legal tradition of the West has its consequences for the
current discussion of the right to die, this ancient tradition is not the only, or even the most important, cultural
force opposed to the right. In fact, as we shall see later,
traditional society in the West was a great deal more hos-
pitable to the right to die than its views on the single subject of suicide would suggest.

A third societal force that often denies the right to
die is the medical profession. Whatever convictions about
dying may prevail in society at large, the patient, after
all, ends up in the hands of a specific profession, with its
own particular ethos. While the physician in the ancient
world was primarily a caretaker of the sick, increasingly the
mission of the modern doctor has shifted from care to cure.
Descriptions of caretaking tend to be pejorative; caretaking
is fit work for handholders and those given to the bedside
manner. Most of the money goes for cure and glamour follows
money. The modern physician has been devoted to the fight
against death. He or she is a member of a resistance movement. Even though other groups in the culture may deviate
from an unconditional fight against death, the physician cannot. His or her patients rely on total dedication. Thus,
the physician would break faith with himself and infect the
professional relationship with distrust if he began to make
decisions about whether to fight for life or hasten death.

A fourth pressure pushing against the right to die is
the spectacular success of modern medical technology. Its
achievements have led increasingly to the exclusive definition of the doctor as fighter. The success of medical technology creates a cultural momentum. It produces a moral
scheme out of the technologist's impulse: what can be done,
should be done. Success inspires the new piety -- not toward
nature, but toward the machine. In the Middle Ages, respect
for the natural impulse to self-preservation led to the opposition to suicide; in recent times, piety toward the machine
argues for the endless prolongation of life. The sheer
existence of the machinery and a team that knows how to use

it argues for its mechanical employment. The machine becomes
<u>autonomous</u>. Instead of serving the life of the patient and
assisting his recovery to permit him once again to serve
others, the machine feeds on the patient. The patient becomes a demonstration of the potency of the machine and the
virtuosity of the medical team. As one resident put it:
"As a university teaching service, we tend to attempt resuscitation on all patients, particularly at the beginning of
the semester" (<u>1</u>).

In the midst of all this enthusiasm, some people feel
that they lose their autonomy and begin to talk much more
passionately than in the past about the right to die. (Their
passion distinguishes them from the Stoics' defense of self-
destruction; Stoics were not supposed to get passionate about
anything -- even suicide.)

A final influence on the question of the right to die is
people's perception of what might be called the metaphysical
pressure in their lives. The destructiveness of disease,
suffering, and death leads victims to enlist the physician as
fighter and provokes in patients and families that terrified
passivity with which they rely on both the physician and
technology. Disease today seems not the absence of positive
powers (sun, food, water, and sleep) but an invasion of
forces that are negative and destructive. Modern people
interpreted disease as an invader with the identification of
bacteria and cancers that wreak havoc in the body. This picture of some diseases dominates the interpretation of all
disease, defines the role of the physician as fighter, and
authorizes appropriations for weapons in the armory of drugs
and procedures with which the professional can wage his war
against disease and death (<u>2</u>). The patient is like Poland
lying helpless between two rival powers that fight out their
battle across relatively defenseless terrain.

Sometimes suffering and death seem a single destructive
experience, at others, the ordeal of suffering becomes distinct from the fear of death. When suffering and death are
experienced as distinctive, the victim tends to develop different ethical responses. Professor Arthur C. McGill, in a
plenary address before the American Academy of Religion,
1974, observed that many movements in ethics can be divided
into those that define absolute evil as death and those that
define it as suffering. If death is the <u>summum malum</u>, then
one is likely to oppose abortion, euthanasia, and war. One
would oppose the right to die. If suffering is the absolute
evil, then one would be willing to pull the plug on an individual life to stop irremediable pain or to risk death in war
rather than face an intolerable slavery (<u>3</u>).

I suspect each group has its own reflexive sense of pre-
eminent good.   When death is perceived as the absolute evil,
life becomes sacred.   When suffering is intolerable, then
wealth, abundance, or quality of life seems more important
than life itself.   Thus the debate gets organized: on one
side -- those who hold to the sanctity of life; on the other
-- those who are more interested in the sanctity of comfort.
One group abhors death and holds life sacred; the other abhors suffering, and prizes quality over life.   Both revere a
creature, not the creator.

My own position on these matters will become clearer as
we proceed.   Suffice it to say at this point that I cannot
wholly side with either party to the debate.   My reluctance
is derived from theological grounds.   These grounds can be
laid out in two ways.

Conventional theological argument begins with a different conception of the sacred than that of either the pro-
lifers or the quality-of-lifers.   Monotheism permits one to
recognize only God as sacred; creatures are good but are not
God; they derive from God.   For this reason the theist cannot subscribe to the slogan of that most famous of the pro-
lifers -- Albert Schweitzer -- Reverence for Life.   (To his
credit, Schweitzer had the courage of his convictions.   Because he was committed to life rather than to quality of
life, he subordinated his dazzling careers as a musician,
composer, philosopher, theologian, and scholar to his voca-
tion as a physician in Lambarene, Africa.)   But neither can
the theist accept the other principle: a reverence for
wealth, which prompts its devotees in the name of quality of
life to deal ruthlessly with the impoverished or the helpless.

This conventional distinction between theism and con-
tending views of the sacred is acceptable enough, but it
does not get at the modern metaphysical problem.   We have already observed that the absorbing modern issue is the problem of evil rather than the definition of good.   The conflicting values of life and quality of life are reflexes
from the deeper apprehensions about the evils of death and
suffering.   Hence the more decisive analysis theologically
requires not the assertion that God transcends the perceived
goods: life and quality of life, but rather that he ultimately encompasses the evils of disease, suffering, and
death.   These evils are real, but not ultimate.   The Christian derives this conclusion from the event at the very center of Christian consciousness: an event in which suffering
and death are not eliminated or repressed but fully exposed.
In the cross, evil exposes itself in its ultimate impotence

to separate man from God. For this reason, men and women
need not cling fiercely to life or quality of life as though
the only alternative to either is absolute nullity.

The Christian theist tradition recognizes that neither
life nor wealth is an absolute good; neither death nor suffering is an absolute evil; that is, powerful enough to deprive human beings of that which is absolutely good. Therefore, the goods and ills we know in life are finally relative; we are free to enjoy goods, but not utterly and irrevocably desolate at their loss, commissioned to resist
evil, but not as though in this resistance alone is our final
resource.

This position would not establish in each case a third
option alongside the other two or guidelines of its own. It
would not always call for a different action, but would open
up a somewhat brighter sky under which to act -- a sky that
has cleared from it the despair of those who believe that
except for life, there is only death, or, except for quality
of life, there is nothing but the final humiliation of pover-
ty. The moral life, by the same token, is not a grim struggle of life against death or "quality of life" against pov-
erty. Neither should our political life be a fierce conflict
of pro-lifers against quality-of-lifers, each heaping epi-
thets on the other, each charging the other with moral blind-
ness. Both positions are ultimately too shrill to reject
their advocate's own excesses: one group clamoring in panic
for life at all costs; the other, proclaiming, give me quality of life or give me (or them) death. A theological perspective suggests that decisions should vary in different
cases: sometimes to relieve suffering, other times to resist death. But in all cases, decisions should not reflect
the pressure of that fear and despair from which absolutism
is often derived.

This position has two general consequences for the medical profession and its use of technology. The profession,
first, ought not to be defined wholly by a fight against
death. When determined exclusively by that fight it presses
for prolongation of life at any cost. The profession should
be free to respond to patients' requests to cease and desist
in the effort to prolong life when it can no longer serve
the health of the host. "Thou shalt not kill, but needst not
strive, officiously, to keep alive." Under some circumstances, the physician engaged in primary care may even be
called upon to find ways (as Eric Cassell has put it) to assist some patients to consent to their own deaths. A physician is not always obligated to fight pneumonia if such
death has become acceptable to the patient, in preference to

death by extraordinarily painful, irreversible and protracted
cancer. There is, after all, a time to live and a time to
die. There is a right to die. Although the progressive im-
poverishment of the patient in dying is not in and of itself
humiliating (the patient may respond to the ordeal with the
dignity of humility rather than humiliation), this impover-
ishment becomes humiliating if it is gratuitously prolonged
by the zeal of others (4).

At the same time, however, neither physicians nor the
society at large ought to prize so highly the quality of life
that they solve the problem of suffering by eliminating the
sufferer. This is often the solution to the problem of evil
propounded by the advocates of active euthanasia. They deny
the capacity to cope with life once terminal pain and suffering have appeared. They assume that life has peaked some-
where on a hill behind them and that all else ahead slopes
downward toward oblivion. They doubt that end-time itself
can be suffused with the human.

With this much in hand, we turn now to distinctions that
are important to discussions of the right to die: 1) between
maximal care and optimal care; 2) between allowing to die and
mercy killing; 3) between euthanasia, passive or active, and
suicide.

1. The basic assumption of an all-out war against death
is that maximal treatment is optimal care. It is doubtful,
however, that maximal medical assault by invasive diagnostic
procedures, by aggressive and complicated drug management, by
enthusiastic cutting and burning, is optimal care for patients. Often such treatment merely distracts from the use
of precious time for what really matters. At worst, the end
result can be somewhat like that Vietnam village that was
destroyed by bombs in the course of being saved. It is salu-
tary, therefore, that two teaching hospitals -- precisely
those institutions which by virtue of resources would be most
tempted to wage all-out war -- have pulled back recently from
total war against death.

The Massachusetts General Hospital has adopted procedures recommended by its Critical Care Committee that would
classify critically ill patients into four groups:

"Class A <u>Maximal</u> <u>therapeutic</u> <u>effort</u> without
          reservation.

Class B <u>Maximal</u> <u>therapeutic</u> <u>effort</u> <u>without</u>
<u>reservation</u> <u>but</u> <u>with</u> <u>daily</u> <u>evalua-</u>
<u>tion</u>.

Class C <u>Selective</u> <u>limitation</u> <u>of</u> <u>therapeutic</u>
<u>measures</u>....A Class C patient is not
an appropriate candidate for admis-
sion to an Intensive Care Unit....

Class D <u>All</u> <u>therapy</u> <u>can</u> <u>be</u> <u>discontinued</u>....
though maximum comfort to the patient
may be continued or instituted...."(<u>5</u>)

The Massachusetts General Hospital (MGH) Report, by implication at least, dissolves two distinctions that previously established for some physicians and moralists clearcut
limits on therapeutic efforts; the distinctions between
starting and stopping machines and between ordinary and
heroic measures. In my judgment, the Report correctly abandons both distinctions for the more apt criterion of the patient's welfare.

a) Physicians commonly feel that they have discretion in
a case only until they start the machines. Once machines are
running, they lose the option of letting the patient die.
This position is understandable psychologically. Once vital
signs have been restored, it seems like killing to pull the
plug. The distinction is misleading, however, in that it
converts a machine from an instrument into a fatality. It
assumes that once the machines are running, they are beyond
the reach of decision-making. They are no longer anyone's
human responsibility. This submissive attitude toward the
equipment repeats the more general submissiveness that the
patient (if competent) and his family feel toward the hospital staff. Once within the precincts of the hospital, the
patient feels that he must comply with its routines and decisions. Like the visitor at the whorehouse, he tends to feel
that he has to go along with what goes on there, once past
the front door.

The MGH Report subordinates the operation of machines to
the patient's welfare as it allows for the reclassification
of patients and provides for daily evaluation of patients in
Class B. The Report also establishes procedures for such
acts as turning off mechanical ventilators at that point in
therapy when the machine may offer maximal treatment but not
optimal care.

b) Similarly the MGH Report implies rejection of the
medical distinction between ordinary and heroic measures;

with the help of this distinction, therapy to prolong life
can be withheld but only if it can be characterized as
heroic. While one may be basically sympathetic to the final
intent of the distinction insofar as it allows some patients
to die, the decision rests too heavily on the status of the
means. If it can be said conscientiously in a given case
that the patient's well-being is best served by the withdrawal of heroic measures, then his welfare may be just as aptly
served by the withdrawal of something as ordinary today as
penicillin.

The MGH Report, in effect, relaxes the distinction between ordinary and heroic when it provides for classification
D, under which all therapy (but not all efforts to provide
comfort) can be discontinued. This distinction could not be
relaxed, of course, unless another criterion took its place
in the light of which therapy is assessed. Professor Paul
Ramsey in his important essay "On (Only) Caring for the Dying," proposed such a criterion: "The right medical practice
will provide those who may get well with the assistance they
need, and it will provide those who are dying with the care
and assistance they need in their final passage. To fail to
distinguish between these two sorts of medical practice would
be to fail to act in accordance with the facts"(6). The crucial distinction does not fall between ordinary and heroic
measures, but between two conditions of patients with two
different sets of needs: those for whom efforts to cure are
appropriate and those for whom efforts at remedy are in vain
but for whom care remains imperative. A given procedure,
whether ordinary or heroic, should be evaluated as to whether
it offers optimal care or merely maximal treatment. The latter may, in fact, neglect the patient, gagging him with the
irrelevant, while denying him what he truly needs.

It may overlook his real condition and wants: "Just as
it would be negligence to the sick to treat them as if they
were about to die, so it is another sort of 'negligence' to
treat the dying as if they are going to get well or might get
well" (7). The MGH Report, with its provision for daily
evaluations, attempts to eliminate the negligence of misplac-
ed treatment.

The MGH guidelines emphasize the needs and welfare of
the patient but pay almost no attention, at least directly,
to the further question of a patient in the process of
decision-making. The guidelines assume that the staff will
make most decisions on behalf of patients. Although the patient and family, along with many other parties, can initi-
ate questions about treatment classification, the final decision rests with the attending physician. Neither the compe-

tent patient nor his or her family has an acknowledged or
regularized place in making those decisions (8). The Report
does not evince that systematic and scrupulous respect for
the competent patient and family that the Beth Israel Hospital of Boston demonstrates in its "Orders Not to Resuscitate"(9).

While declaring that the hospital's general policy is
"to act affirmatively to preserve the life of all patients,"
the Beth Israel document acknowledges those situations in
which heroic measures "might be both medically unsound and so
contrary to the patient's wishes or expectations as not to be
justified." The document then establishes procedures by
which the competent patient (or family, in the case of an incompetent patient) can collaborate in a standing order not to
resuscitate -- specifically, in those cases that satisfy the
conditions of irreversibility, irreparability, and imminence
of death.

On the negative side, the Beth Israel document deals
only with orders not to resuscitate. It thus operates too
restrictively within the old distinctions between starting
and stopping the machines and between ordinary and heroic
measures. It does not deal with that more extended range of
cases in which it may be appropriate for the patient's welfare to stop (and not just not start) procedures or even to
stop procedures that are less than heroic.

On the positive side, the document tackles head-on the
consent issue, the question of a patient's rights. This issue, however, is deeper than the formal question of patient
freedom; that is, the question as to whether patients or
physicians shall have the final decision as to when and for
what reasons efforts to prolong life shall cease. To be
sure, human dignity is at stake if patients are categorically
denied the liberty to participate in decisions having to do
with themselves, but dignity in this particular case, if it
is actually to be exercised under the conditions of <u>informed</u>
consent, rests on a deeper dignity; that is, the capacity of
patients to cope with their own dying. Much well-intentioned
medical practice is guided by the conviction that the liberty
to cope with one's own dying is an unwanted liberty. The
physician, for example, who brought the series of articles in
<u>The New England Journal of Medicine</u> to my attention was skep-
tical about the readiness of patients to participate in decisions about their own dying. He commented candidly that he
"liked" the Report of the Massachusetts General Hospital, but
found the "other" policy statement that sought patient concurrence in such matters ghoulish. His judgment reflects a
widely shared skepticism about the likelihood that patients

will find it a favor to be confronted with the question of
their courage in the face of death. Informed consent remains
"pro forma" if the patient is unwilling to face his own dying. He signs the papers quickly because he is disinclined
to entertain the prospect of a medical failure. The issue of
informed consent poses at the deepest level the question of
the human possibility for dignity, humility, and courage in
facing death; the problem, ultimately, of consent to one's
own dying. At its deepest level, the question of the right
to die springs from the duty to die well.

2.   Some moralists, like Joseph Fletcher, believe that
the distinction between allowing to die and mercy killing is
hypocritical quibbling over technique. They are disposed to
call "allowing to die" passive euthanasia and mercy killing
active euthanasia and collapse the distinction between the
two. Since the consequences are the same -- whether the patient dies by acts of omission or commission -- what matters
the route the patient took there? By either procedure he
ends up dead.

Other moralists, opposed to active euthanasia, believe
that the distinction between allowing to die and mercy killing is worth preserving and in favor of the former. This
position can be defended in two ways, either by exploring the
obligations of the community to the dying or by examining the
rights (and, for some religious traditions, the duties) of
the dying. Most opponents of active euthanasia begin with
the obligations of the community, particularly those of medical professionals. Professor Ramsey, as we have seen, has
defined that professional obligation as the mandate to give
care. This imperative sets a limit on the efforts to prolong
the process of dying. It justifies allowing to die. There
comes a time when physicians, family, and friends must cease
and desist, not in order to abandon the patient, but to provide for care and only care. Otherwise treatment is mis-
directed and ultimately negligent. Professor Ramsey, however, would not extend the mandate of care to mercy killing.
To care in the form of killing is to defect from the obligation by eliminating the patient to whom care is directed.
While the irreversibly dying live, they claim from us care
and not something else -- neither officious efforts to prolong their lives nor short cuts to end them. Mercy killing
is impatient with the patient. In its own inverted way it
abandons him.

Since Professor Ramsey bases his rejection of active
euthanasia on the imperative to care, rather than on the absolute sacredness of life, he must concede, at least theo-
retically, two special circumstances under which mercy kill-

ing might be permissible: when the patient is in a permanent
comatose state so profound as to be totally inaccessible to
human care or when the dying patient experiences extreme and
unendurable pain for which no relief can be offered.
(Whether in fact any patients satisfy either of these conditions is a determination which only the competent physician
[and not the moralist] can make; and even physicians, if the
reports of the staff at St. Christopher's Hospice can be
credited, have failed to explore fully the degree to which
pain can be held at bay.) Under these very limited conditions, active euthanasia may be allowable to, but never obligatory upon, the professional. The right to die, therefore,
reaches its acceptable limit in the negative right, as Professor James Childress has put it, of "not having one's dying
process extended or interfered with." The proponents of
active euthanasia push on to the more positive claim "to have
others help one to become dead." The right to die passes
over into the right to be killed with serious negative consequences (argues Professor Childress in an unpublished paper
on "To Kill or Let Die") for the trust between doctor and patient upon which the professional relationship depends.

The so-called "death with dignity" movement attempts to
specify contractually those conditions under which a patient
may be allowed to die without compromising the obligation of
the community to care. This group proposes that a patient
reach an agreement with his or her physician concerning those
circumstances (terminal and irreversible) under which one
would want life-supporting systems withdrawn.

So far so good. I do, however, have a caveat to offer
on the subject. The term "death with dignity" should not be
restricted to the contractual freedom to choose the time of
one's own dying. While it may include that, it needs to include much more than that if this freedom is to be protected.

The decision of a patient to instruct his or her physician to pull the plug is not a dignified decision if it is
humanly or financially coerced. The decision becomes forced
when the society devotes too much money to glamourous techniques for the prolongation of life at the expense of humane
care for the dying. Under these circumstances, an individual
may have only a forced choice between inhuman prolongation
versus a rapid termination of his life. He needs also the
third option of an environment of dignified care.

Put another way, dying with dignity (in the sense of the
rapid termination of life) requires, if it is to be an uncoerced decision, protecting the dignity of dying itself.
This, in turn, requires caring for the dying with dignity and

this will not occur unless we respect the dignity of caring for the dying. Adequate social support is required for systems and professions concerned with care, if there is to be real freedom in the choice not to avail oneself further of the opportunity for care.|

To put it bluntly -- if a member of the middle class instructs his doctor under certain conditions to withdraw procedures the result of which is to bring about death, we can be reasonably sure of the uncoerced nature of his decision. By virtue of finances he has available resources to secure a level of care beyond minimal standards. But others less fortunate than he may be driven to a decision to terminate because the care of the dying is so poor. Their only available solution is to terminate life as quickly as possible. The poor should not be made an offer which they cannot afford to decline because the current alternative for living is unacceptable.

Very practically, then, the right to die must be protected from abuse but its placement within the larger context of the right to equal access to life and health care. Death with dignity is too narrowly defined if it simply places within my reach the chance to get out of a miserable life. The movement may even be pernicious if it decreases within the society the motivation to provide humane care.

In a large city in another country, there is a road called "The Street of the Good Death". The street is so called because of an exceptionally fine hospital located there. The hospital, however, is noted neither for its life-prolonging equipment not for its readiness to put to sleep its inmates but for its provision of good care for the dying. Euthanasia happens to be the name of that street.

A somewhat less conventional way of approaching the distinction between allowing to die and mercy killing is to focus on the obligations not of the community but of the dying. With the exception of the Roman Catholic tradition in moral theology, modern teachers in the field of medical ethics are almost mute on the subject. The reason for this silence lies in the somewhat selective appropriation today of the ancient religious tradition of the West. In a secular age, we are disposed to retain a remnant of the ethic of love (translated into medical ethics as the obligation of the community to care) but we know little of the ancient ethic of humility and patience, virtues which the patient may need when care has done all it can. Modern Western Protestant Christianity and secular humanism which has been its offshoot has been almost exclusively committed to the virtue of love rather than the

virtue of humility, to the dynamics of giving rather than the
more difficult art of receiving. The sick are distressed.
What is more natural than to respond to their distress with
the works of charity? Give them what they need, and since
they can apparently be given more in a hospital, put them
there and put them in the hands of professionals who are expert givers.

Well and good, but we are almost totally silent on the
subject of the virtues of the patient. Medical ethics con-
centrates exclusively on the ethics of the expert, the master giver. The subtlest dehumanization of the patient may
occur in that we do not take seriously the question of his
virtues and vices,·the nobility or the meanness of his responses to his condition. We act and reflect as though the
patient does not have a moral life. The virtues of patience
and courage may be as important to death with dignity as an
environment of care. Sometimes the strongest response to the
humiliation of illness is not loving care, but the patient's
own humility. Moreover, as we take seriously the moral role
of the patient, we may begin to see that the physician re-
ceives from, as well as gives to, his patients and that
humility may be an unexpected ingredient in professional
life.

It is impossible to discuss today the question of the
patient and his responsibilities without reckoning with the
concept of a good death. To its credit, the euthanasia movement has reintroduced the patient into the discussion of
medical ethics because it poses the question of a good death.
This question, however, will have to be discussed in historical perspective because Western society appears to have experienced a major change in its conception of a good death.

Most modern people equate a good death with a sudden
death. They want to go quickly in an accident; they prefer
a heart attack to cancer. To the best of my knowledge,
Soren Kierkegaard of the nineteenth century was the first to
draw attention to the modern preference for a sudden death
(10). (Ironically, the modern world has produced simul-
taneously a desire for a sudden death and the incredibly expensive C-T Scanner, a half million dollar early warning system about diseases largely irremediable!) The preference
has become so widespread today that almost any other choice
seems incomprehensible. If, of course, any other choice is
truly unintelligible, then one would be more inclined to collapse the distinction between active and passive euthanasia
and go the quickest route possible.

Yet historically, it would appear, another preference is possible. We know, for example, that people in the Middle Ages preferred some advance warning about their death. They listed a sudden death among the many evils from which devout folk should pray for deliverance. Clearly, a warning is desirable if people feel that they have some way of preparing for an event. The housewife deems it unfortunate when a guest catches her in hair curlers without something in the pantry. She prefers a little warning so that she can rise to the occasion. The traditional prayers of the church concerning death acknowledged a link between warning and preparation. The Rogation Day list of evils from which the believer prayed for deliverance included the evil of a <u>sudden</u> and <u>unprovided for</u> death. Conversely, a good death included warning and very specific preparations.

Medieval literature was filled with premonitions of death (<u>11</u>). The customary phrase was "his time has come." After forewarning, the dying man or woman made preparations. First, the dying person might adopt prescribed gestures or postures: sometimes the head oriented to the East, the hands crossed, or the face turned up to heaven. Preparations included, second, the important business of going through the experiences of grief and reconciliation with relatives, companions, and helpers. Grief occurred on both sides. Those about to be bereaved needed to express their grief over imminent loss, and the dying man needed to grieve over the loss of his world. Such mourning was short-lived but not to be denied or obscured. Some measure of suffering was an acceptable part of human dying. The further work of preparation included the reconciliation of the dying man or woman with companions and friends. Finally, the dying person uttered prayers of confession and petition, followed by the only specifically ecclesiastical part of the occasion, the prayers of absolution by the priest.

Where did all this work of preparation take place? In the bedchamber of the dying. We must remember, moreover, that the bedroom was not on this occasion a <u>private</u> room. "The dying man's bedchamber became a public place to be entered freely" by relatives, friends, servants, and children. Only in the eighteenth century, with medical concern for hygiene, did doctors begin to isolate the dying person in his bedroom. Thenceforward dying became a secret act.

Until the last two hundred years dying was a public ceremony; but who organized this ceremony? As Ariès points out: The dying person himself functioned as the master of ceremonies.

How did he learn to do it? Very simply. As a child he had seen others accept responsibility for their own dying. He had not been excluded from the room. He knew the protocol. He would do it in turn when his own time had come. "Thus, death was familiar and near, evoking no great awe or fear." That is why Ariès characterizes this whole period as living and dying with a sense of "tamed death."

The contrast today is striking. Instead of dying at home in one's own bedchamber, 80% of Americans die in a hospital or in a nursing home. Earlier, dying was a public ceremony witnessed by a company including relatives, helpers, friends, and children. But today, death often comes, even for those who have families, secretly in the hospital, unwatched except at a technical level by the all-monitoring eye of a cardiac machine. If the patient were to meet death heroically, only the machine would know it.

"A visitor to a hospital can often spot a room where a terminally ill patient is being treated. It's usually, if not invariably, dark. The shades are always pulled down, the draperies are closed, the people speak softly -- if at all. There's often a physical withdrawal from the dying patient's bed" (12).

Finally, in earlier centuries, the person dying organized himself for the event with some sense of protocol. Today, however, others manage dying. We call it management of the terminally ill. A new specialist has been added to interpret and handle the event: the thanatologist. "So live that when thy thanatologist comes...." Still another specialist looms on the horizon, the dolorist. Generally, though, machines take charge; relatives and friends must give them berth; and hospital attendants are their acolytes. Death has become a mechanical process. The person has been robbed of his own dying; and if you add to theft the ignorance in which he is often kept, he loses what earlier cultures felt to be important to a good death -- the forewarning that invited one not simply to participate in medical decisions but to prepare and to take over one's own dying.

Perhaps it is clear now why one must be hesitant about judging earlier Western culture, on the question of its attitude toward the right to die, entirely on the basis of its opposition to suicide: it may have been opposed to suicide, but it was not opposed to the right to die. In fact, it fully expected a person to reckon with, and to govern his own dying. The age acknowledged that not all suffering is utterly inhuman; dependency, abhorrent. Although it is wrong to sentimentalize suffering or to romanticize death and dying, it is equally wrong to assume that men and women cannot be human in the midst of suffering and death, that they have no role to play in the face of dependency, no virtues to evince.

Modern culture, to the contrary, not only denies the right to die by its often mindless prolongation of life, but, just as seriously, denies with the same heedlessness the right of the person to do his own dying. Since modern procedures, moreover, have made dying at the hands of the experts and the machines a prolonged and painful business, emotionally and financially as well as physically, they have built up pressure behind the euthanasia movement which asserts, not the right to die, but the right to be killed.

The basic thrust of the euthanasia movement is to engineer death rather than to face dying. Euthanasia would bypass dying to get one dead as quickly as possible. It proposes to relieve suffering by knocking out the interval between the two states, living and dead. The emotional impulse behind the movement is understandable in an age when dying is made such an inhumanly endless business. The movement opposes the horrors of a purely technical death by using technique to eliminate the victim. The alternative I have outlined argues, at least in principle, that warning can provoke good; that with forewarning and time for preparation, reconciliation can take place; and that advance grieving by those about to be bereaved may ease their pain. Some psychiatrists have observed that those bereaved who lost someone accidentally have a more difficult time recovering from the loss than those who have suffered through a period of illness before the death. Those who have lost a close relative by accident are more likely to experience what Geoffrey Gorer has called limitless grief. The community, moreover, needs its aged and dependent, its sick and its dying, and the virtues which they sometimes evince -- the virtues of humility, courage, and patience -- just as much as the community needs the virtues of justice and love manifest in the agents of its care. Thus, on the whole, I am in favor of social policy that would take seriously the notion of allowing to die, rather than killing for mercy, that is, which would recognize that moment in illness when it is no longer meaningful to bend every effort to cure or to prolong life and when it is fitting to allow patients to do their own dying. This policy seems most consonant with the obligations of the community to care and the patient to finish his course.

3. Does the right to die extend to the right to suicide? Clearly not without a distinction. Allowing to die and mercy killing normally cover cases in which the patient is manifestly and imminently dying from a disease the course

of which is physically irreversible. The suicide is not necessarily, or even usually, dying. Further, the responses of allowing to die and mercy killing usually apply to patients who move toward a state into which care cannot reach. The suicide may suffer; and his isolation is often such that he does not receive or accept care. But, physically at least and psychologically perhaps, his pain and suffering could be relieved; he is accessible to care. Do professionals, friends, and relatives therefore have an obligation, protestations to the contrary, to preserve life? A concluding comment on this limited aspect of suicide is in order.

Several considerations argue for intervention. a) Although life is not an absolute, it is a fundamental good. b) The impulse to suicide is often transient yet the act has irreversible consequences. A given intervention may not always prevent a future successful attempt at suicide but it will assure at least that the eventual deed is deliberate or compulsive (rather than merely impulsive). c) The fact that suicide usually has destructive consequences for survivors argues against it. d) Since the ratio of attempted to successful suicides is 8:1 or 10:1, the act must be interpreted at the least as ambivalent. Occasionally an unsuccessful suicide may result from incompetence; usually, however, it is, in the common parlance, a "cry for help." If this is so, then the medical profession, friends, and relatives fail in their duties if they refuse to respond.

One exception and one qualification need to be considered: so-called rational suicide is the exception. It results neither from biological/emotional problems or from fateful circumstances but rather from a philosophical conviction -- debatable, to be sure, with respect to the status of the right, but nevertheless rationalized and determined. One might want to argue with such a person, but one should not forcibly prevent him from committing the act or punish him should, through some fluke, it be unsuccessful in its outcome.

The "cry for help" argument needs interpretation and leads to a qualification. I would prefer to substitute the phrase, "a cry for a change." A "cry for help" signals that the would-be suicide basically wants to be relieved of his suicide impulse and get a little attention. Suicide prevention operating at this level does not go deep enough. It merely resists suicide but seems to have no better plan than to put the suicide back into the same old box, this time relieved of his impulse to get out of the box because he has gotten the attention he wants.

Why, however, has the suicide cried for help in the peculiar way that he has? Because he is crying for a peculiar
kind of help, that is, help that will bring an utterly radical change in his life. Attempted suicide is a violent
statement of the wish for a change, a declaration that describes the change in the most radical of terms -- a change
from life to death.

The suicide wishes for, in James Hillman's phrase (13),
the experience of death -- the death of his old life. He has
no appetite for a return to his former existence, superfi-
cially divested of the impulse to die. He wants to die, he
needs to die to his former life and come into a new life. He
needs to go through a death experience, that is, a total and
radical transformation of himself. He wishes for a sea-
change in the very depths of his being. Thus mere suicide
prevention is not enough help for those whose will to die is
a haunted expression of the will to live abundantly.

NOTES

1. See Diana Crane, The Sanctity of Social Life: Physicians' Treatment of Criticially Ill Patients (New York: Russell Sage Foundation, 1975).

2. For this more demonic and melodramatic interpretation of disease, see René Dubos, The Mirage of Health, ch. on "Aesculapius and Hygeia" (New York: Harper & Row, 1971); Arthur C. McGill, Suffering: A Test of Theological Method, ch. 2, "Demonism: the Spiritual Reality of Our Age" (Philadelphia: Geneva Press, 1966); and Ivan Illych, Medical Nemesis (New York: Pantheon Books, 1976).

3. It is doubtful whether the perception of death or suffering as absolute evil controls ethical decisions consistently and deductively in all areas. I would be surprised, e.g., if pro-lifers were invariably opponents of the Vietnam War.

4. Recall, for instance, Chevy Chase's news bulletins on the struggle to keep Generalissimo Franco alive. Life-prolongation extended beyond the humiliating to the ridiculous.

5. "Optimum Care for Hopelessly Ill Patients; A Report of the Clinical Care Committee of the Massachusetts General Hospital," The New England Journal of Medicine 295:7 (Aug. 12, 1976), 362-64.

6. Paul Ramsey, The Patient as Person (New Haven: Yale University Press, 1970), p. 133.

7. Ibid., p. 133. Professor Ramsey exercises care to show how some Roman Catholic moralists (e.g., Fr. Gerald Kelly, S.J.) have taken steps, albeit cautious, in the direction of his views. Physicians tend to distinguish between ordinary and heroic measures, on the basis of the status of the means used. Recent interpreters of the Roman Catholic distinction between ordinary and extraordinary means are more inclined to include the condition of the patient and not just the status of the means as factors in decision-making. Although his remarks are carefully hedged, Fr. Kelly recognizes circumstances under which a means as ordinary as water may be inappropriate. For this reason, my criticisms in this section have been chiefly directed against the distinction made by the medical community.

8. The single exception is the requirement that the physician consult with and secure the concurrence of the family in the decision to perform certain acts of commission (such as turning off a mechanical ventilator on a patient) that will lead to death.

9. Mitchell T. Rabkin, M.D., Gerald Gillerman, J.D., and Nancy R. Rice, J.D., "Orders Not to Resuscitate," The New England Journal of Medicine, op. cit., pp. 364-66.

10. See his Thoughts on Crucial Situations in Life (Minneapolis: Augsburg Publishing House, 1941).

11. For what follows, see Philippe Ariès, Western Attitudes Towards Death (Baltimore: Johns Hopkins Press, 1974).

12. Donald Kimetz, M.D., Louisville Courier Journal, Feb. 10, 1976.

13. James Hillman, Suicide and the Soul (New York: Harper & Row, 1964), ch. 4.

Demands for Life
and Requests for Death:
The Judicial Dilemma

Leslie S. Rothenberg

"Judges are not essentially different from
other government officials. Fortunately they
remain human even after assuming their judicial
duties." (1)

Much of the literature which has emerged during the last decade on the topic of death and
dying has focused on the experience of patients,
families of patients, and physicians in their
acceptance or denial of the inevitability of death.

The purpose of this paper is to briefly explore the attitudes of judges regarding their own
roles as decision-makers in cases involving the
assertion of a right to die. In such professional
contexts, judges confront the same issues of life
and death as do patients, family members, and
physicians; the difference is that judges may use
the awesome power of the government to enforce
their decisions. For that reason, it seems strange
that greater attention has not been previously
paid to judicial attitudes and their relationship,
if any, to the outcome of "right to die" cases
brought to the courts.

Perhaps one explanation for the lack of prior
study of these attitudes is the admitted difficulty
of collecting reliable data. Judges, even more
than most other persons, find it undesirable in
their professional roles to articulate their personal feelings or attitudes about the facts presented to them.

The _persona_ or mask of the judge is impersonal
neutrality with a corresponding exaltation of

rationality and intellect. John Noonan has
described the accepted rationale for this mask in
his insightful study of persons and masks of the
law:

> The paradigmatic form of law, trial
> in court, reinforces the necessity to
> exalt the role of rule. In the paradigm,
> the judge hears conflicting parties and
> decides upon the evidence which they
> present. The evidence is related to
> his decision through his selection of a
> rule. If the judge looks at who the
> parties are, he is not looking at the
> evidence. A judge who takes into account
> who the parties are will favor one or the
> other. A biased judge is no judge at all.

> If the judge looks at the rules, he
> is acting in accordance with the paradigm,
> which requires two persons to be in con-
> troversy, and a third person, who prefers
> neither, to decide. The judge indicates
> his impartiality, he proves his good
> faith, by looking not at the persons but
> at the rule. The rule is neutral, "above"
> the contestants and the judge. (2)

As if to reinforce this paradigm, several
judges (3) have chosen to quote Justice Benjamin
N. Cardozo's classic work, The Nature of Judicial
Process,(4) by way of warning against undue
judicial intervention in right to die matters. The
judge, Cardozo wrote,

> even when he is free, is still not
> wholly free. He is not to innovate
> at pleasure. He is not a knight-
> errant roaming at will in pursuit of
> his own ideal of beauty or of goodness.
> He is to draw his inspiration from
> consecrated principles. He is not to
> yield to spasmodic sentiment, to vague
> and unregulated benevolence. He is to
> exercise a discretion informed by tra-
> dition, methodized by analogy, disciplin-
> ed by system, and subordinated to "the
> primordian necessity of order in the
> social life."(5)

Not surprisingly, these same judges fail to
mention Cardozo's equally strong admonition not to
forget human emotions and drives which influence
and shape the judicial process. Suggesting that
these human elements are rarely discussed because
judges fear they might "lose respect and confidence
by the reminder that they are subject to human
limitations," Cardozo pointed out that judges like
to think of the judicial process as "coldly objective and impersonal."(6)

This mask of impersonality seldom yields articulated feelings or attitudes in published judicial
opinions, and thus, when examining decisions in
the right to die area, a reader is struck by the
occasional lowering of the mask and the revelation
of personal discomfort (even anguish) and ambivalence on the part of the judge deciding the case.
The remainder of this paper will be devoted to an
examination of such reactions, followed by a proposal to relieve judges, partially at least, of
this burden in future right to die cases that are
presented to their courts.

Given the looseness with which the term,
"ambivalence," has been used lately, a definitional
digression seems appropriate. Ambivalence has
been characterized by William Winslade as the co-
existence in the same person of "unresolved conflicting feelings which are strong and long-last,
ing, concerning matters of importance, and have a
significant impact upon the person."(7) Typically,
ambivalence is felt towards some object which has
great importance for the person concerned; issues
of life and death are often subject to it.(8)
Choosing to define it as "the simultaneous attract-
ion toward and repulsion from a single object,
person or action,"(9) thanatologist Edwin
Shneidman has observed that ambivalence is "the
most important psychodynamic concept to grasp if
we are to understand our attitudes toward
death." (10)

Because persons torn by ambivalence are
likely to be indecisive,(11) and because indecis-
ion, or the suggestion of such, is anathema to the
judge as professional decision-maker, we are unlikely to find clear-cut evidence of ambivalence
in published judicial opinions. If we were to
imagine how judicial ambivalence might show itself,

we might develop language not unlike that which
Professor Lon Fuller of the Harvard Law School put
in the mouth of a mythical appellate judge in his
famous hypothetical case of the Speluncean
Explorers.(12) This imaginary criminal case, known
to many law students who have struggled with its
implications, involves four men who are imprisoned
in a cave and find it necessary for survival-
purposes to kill a fifth companion and eat his
flesh on the twenty-third day of their imprison-
ment. They are subsequently indicted and convicted
for murder and are sentenced to hang. They appeal
their case to a mythical appellate court, and
Fuller has one of the justices express not only his
ambivalence, but also the extent to which he is
unable to subordinate his emotional reaction to a
more typically intellectual and rational consideration of the legal rules:

> In the discharge of my duties as a justice
> of this court I am usually able to dissociate
> the emotional and intellectual sides of my
> reactions, and to decide the case before
> me entirely on the basis of the latter.
> In passing on this tragic case I find
> that my usual resources fail me. On the
> emotional side I find myself torn between
> sympathy for these men and a feeling of
> abhorrence and disgust at the monstrous
> act they committed. I had hoped that I
> should be able to put these contradictory
> emotions to one side as irrelevant, and
> to decide the case on the basis of a
> convincing and logical demonstration of
> the result demanded by our law. Unfor-
> tunately, this deliverance has not
> been vouchsafed me. (13)

It is this ambivalence that occurs when adversa-
ries, in a courtroom setting, raise seemingly
contradictory priorities of prolonging life and
allowing death--the classic right to die case--which
we must now examine.

Many of the judicial decisions raising issues
of the choice between life and death have involved
the refusal, often--but not necessarily--on
religious grounds, to consent to medical treatment.
One case to which judges, who find themselves involved with "right to die" issues, have often
looked for guidance involved a 25-year-old mother,

a Jehovah's Witness. (14) Brought into Georgetown
Hospital in 1963 with a ruptured ulcer and having
lost two-thirds of her body's blood supply, the
woman and her husband both refused to permit a
blood transfusion. Such medical treatment, they
indicated, would violate their religious beliefs
as Jehovah's Witnesses. When death seemed imminent
unless a blood transfusion was administered, the
hospital sought the assistance of their lawyers,
who applied to the District Court in Washington for
permission to give the transfusion. District Judge
Edward A. Tamm denied the application, and the
lawyers immediately sought the assistance of an
appellate judge, J. Skelly Wright, who is a judge
of the District of Columbia Circuit of the U. S.
Court of Appeals. Judge Wright went to the hospital, spoke with the patient, her husband and
several doctors. When the patient's husband, after
much discussion, refused to authorize the transfusion, Judge Wright signed an order allowing for
such transfusions as the doctors decided were
necessary to save her life. (15)

    In justifying his actions, Judge Wright first
argued that this was the kind of a case that courts
were suppose to decide, and that it involved an
issue of the patient's--and the hospital's--rights
which he felt the legislature was unlikely to
resolve. "Courts sit to decide such questions," he
wrote. (16). Worth noting is the fact that Judge
Wright happens to be a devoutly religious person,
and Georgetown College (now Georgetown University)
happens to be a religiously-affiliated institution.
But in his explanation in granting the order
(technically known as an "emergency writ"), Judge
Wright spoke not of his personal beliefs, but of
his sense of being compelled by the factual circumstances in which

    a life hung in the balance. There was no
    time for research and reflection. Death
    could have mooted the case in a matter
    of minutes, if action were not taken to
    preserve the status quo. To refuse to
    act, only to find later that the law
    required action, was a risk I was unwill-
    ing to accept. I determined to act on the
    side of life. (17)

The patient survived and made a request,

through her lawyer, for a rehearing of the legal
issues involved by all nine judges sitting on the
District of Columbia Court of Appeals. Her petition
was denied, (18) but three judges were openly
critical of Judge Wright's action in signing the
order to authorize the transfusions. The best-
known of the three now serves as the Chief Justice
of the United States, Chief Justice Warren Burger.

Serving at the time as a Circuit Judge, Judge
Burger analyzed the case in great detail, pointing
out the difficulties for judges to decide questions
perplexing physicians, philosophers and theologians.
He repeated the·quotation from Justice Cardozo
given above and emphasized the need for judges to
be aware of the limits of their power which, he
said, "is simply an acknowledgement of human
fallibility." (19). In conclusion, he wrote that
judges must accept that there are many problems
which judges cannot solve, and that "this is as it
should be." (20)

> Some matters of essentially private
> concern and others of enormous public
> concern, are beyond the reach of judges.(21)

While Judge Burger's dissent in this case, based
on judicial restraint, is rarely quoted or remembered, many judges are familiar with Judge Wright's
action and clearly approve of it.

In a 1965 case (22) in the United States
District Court in New Haven, Connecticut, District
Judge Robert C. Zampano cited Wright's action as
precedent for granting a request by a Veterans
Administration Hospital to order that blood transfusions be administered to a 39-year-old father,
also a Jehovah's Witness, who was suffering from a
bleeding ulcer. Judge Zampano went further than
Judge Wright in saying that he would not permit
the patient to "demand mistreatment," by which he
meant asking the doctors involved to violate their
own conscience. (23) Judge Zampano, however,
makes no mention of his own feelings or attitudes
about the case in his written opinion.

In that same year, in a New York State court,
another trial court judge, Supreme Court Justice
Jacob Markowitz, was faced with a similar request.
(24)

A woman who had suffered extensive bleeding following a caesarian section refused to consent to a
blood transfusion because of her beliefs as a
Jehovah's Witness. The mother of six children
whose family unsuccessfully begged her to allow the
transfusion, the patient was diagnosed as critically ill and placed on the hospital's "danger
list." (25) Her husband, with the aid of the Legal
Aid Society, sought an order from Justice Markowitz
similar to the one that had been granted in the
earlier case by Judge Wright and District Judge
Zampano. Justice Markowitz gave such an order,
but not without much soul-searching. Fortunately
for our purposes, he expressed his concerns in his
written opinion.

First, he acknowledged that this case "generated a barrage of legal niceties, misinformation and
emotional feelings on the part of all concerned--
including the court personnel." (26). Nobody
questioned whether this was an appropriate case for
a court to decide, he wrote, nor could he forget
his own convictions with regard to the individual's
right to be left alone as well as the fact that a
human life "hung in the balance." (27) Having
said that much, he revealed his own sense of personal anguish as the decision-maker:

> Never before had my judicial robe weighed
> so heavily on my shoulders. Years of
> legal training, experience and respon-
> sibility had added a new dimension to
> my mental processes--I, almost by
> reflex action, subjected the papers
> to the test of justiciability, jurisdic-
> tion and legality. I read [the Georgetown
> case decided by Judge Wright] and was
> convinced of the proper course from a
> legal standpoint. Yet, ultimately, my
> decision to act to save this woman's
> life was rooted in more fundamental
> precepts. (28)

Worried about "how legalistic minded our
society has become," Justice Markowitz concluded
his opinion by describing the factor that he
found most personally compelling in this case:

> I was reminded of "The Fall" by Camus,
> and I knew that no release--no legalistic

        absolution--would absolve me or the
        Court from responsibility if, I,
        speaking for the Court, answered
        "No" to the question "Am I my
        brother's keeper?" This woman wanted
        to live. I could not let her die! (29)

     The mask of impersonality, the persona of
neutral objectivity, is altogether dropped.
Justice Markowitz reveals his innermost torment;
he then resolves his ambivalence by deciding, as
did Judge Wright, that the patient "really" wants
to live but cannot authorize the transfusions and
makes the decision in favor of life.

     There was no procedural need for this display
of human emotion and feeling. Justice Markowitz
could have simply cited the Georgetown case and
indicated that his order was thus legally justified. A Long Island judge, Justice Mario Pittoni,
who was also sitting on the state trial court
(confusingly named the "Supreme Court;" the highest court in New York is known as the "Court of
Appeals"), had done exactly that a year earlier in
signing an order permitting a surgical operation
for a comatose patient who was critically ill and
whose wife refused to give her consent. No
personal feelings, no human emotions, just a
matter-of-record statement of the pertinent facts
and the law.(30) But Justice Markowitz wasn't
content to hide his human struggle behind the
opaque folds of his judicial robe. Again, perhaps
by coincidence, he holds strong religious beliefs,
and when he was unfortunate enough to have yet
another case of this same genre presented to him
nine months later, he was determined to deal
directly with this issue of judicial decision-
making and its propriety in such cases.

     The second case (31) presented an unusual set
of facts. Two of the three children of an 80-year-
old woman patient petitioned the Court for an order
permitting an amputation of their mother's right
ankle and foot. Both of these two children were
lawyers practicing together in the same law office,
and they handled the legal proceedings by and for
themselves. The patient's third son was a physician, and it was his refusal to consent to the
operation--as one of the next of kin--that
precipitated the legal proceedings.

Justice Markowitz determined that the patient
had a history of arteriosclerotic heart disease and
diabetes, and had suffered three strokes and the
same number of attacks of pneumonia. Gangrene had
set in around her right foot and heel, and her
physician stated that an operation was urgently
needed and was a matter of life and death.(32)
After appointing a psychiatrist to examine the
patient and to determine whether she had sufficient
mental capacity to sign the consent forms herself,
Justice Markowitz learned not only that the
psychiatrist believed her to be legally incapable
of giving an informed consent to the operation, but
also that the patient, whether competent or not to
make such decisions, didn't want an amputation.
Furthermore, he was informed that there was no
assurance that the amputation would be effective;
that, in the opinion of several other physicians,
there was no medical emergency; and that both the
Court-appointed guardian for the patient and the
Court-appointed psychiatrist did not believe that
the Court should authorize the operation. (33)

Armed with this seemingly helpful information,
the judge then commented:

> Thus, it becomes apparent that this
> proceeding, where responsible members
> of a family, including a physician-
> son, unfortunately cannot agree on what
> is medically necessary or proper for
> their aged and infirm mother, presents
> an example of a grave dilemma which
> confronts those who engage in the heal-
> ing arts, and on the other hand, some
> basic fundamental issues on the nature
> and scope of judicial power and the
> wisdom or propriety of judicial interven-
> tion. (34)

There was clearly a difference of opinion
among the doctors as to the advisability of the amputation (only one of three doctors favoring it),
and the physician-son of the patient stated to
Justice Markowitz that "assaultive surgery in a
terminal case in the name of emergency is cruelty
beyond description."(35)

Justice Markowitz openly complained that this
legal proceeding was necessitated only by the

doctor's fear of civil liability if they proceeded
without proper consent. He saw this as an improper
shifting of the burden of the physicians' medical
responsibilities to the courts.(36) More importantly, however, the judge posed a fundamental
question of the propriety of judicial action in
such cases:

> However, from the frequently recurring
> applications to the courts in instances
> similar to the case at bar, it is evident
> that in the absence of protective legis-
> lation, members of the medical profession,
> by their repeated insistence upon a written
> release in any and all cases prior to
> operative procedures, in effect, compel
> judicial intervention in matters when the
> necessity or value of a legal opinion
> alone is highly questionable. Confronted
> by a situation such as this, I am of the
> opinion that the time has come for courts
> to inquire where a continued condonation
> of such action and where a continued assump-
> tion of jurisdiction over such matters
> lead. Undoubtedly, physicians, surgeons
> and hospitals, like judges, lawyers and
> others as well, are often faced with
> seemingly irreconcilable demands and
> conflicting pressures. Philosophers and
> theologians have pondered these problems,
> and, as is to be expected, different
> groups evolved different solutions.
> Religious beliefs and doctrines, for example,
> complicated equitable solutions sought by
> courts in blood tranfusions cases...(37)

Having raised the question, Justice Markowitz
then proceeded to provide his own answers: namely,
that a courtroom is not a proper place, and a legal
proceeding is not the proper vehicle, to decide
such questions. (38) Yet still concerned about his
role, he continued further:

> It is regrettable that the court here
> is placed in the position of refusing,
> or what to many may seem the refusal,
> to act in order to save a life or to
> ameliorate suffering. The contrary is
> the fact. It is because of the court's
> deep concern for Mrs. Nemser's life and

well-being that it is reminding those
whose responsibility it actually is,
to act appropriately, not arbitrarily
and without fear. (39)

Finally, having decided the case by denying
the requested order, Justice Markowitz suggested

that an appropriate study should be made
by members of the legal and medical
professions, hospital personnel, and
the community in general, including its
spiritual advisers, to consider problems
akin to those raised by this application.
Certainly the social aspects of such
problems far outweigh their legal
implications.(40)

There have, of course, been other similar
cases. In Florida, Judge David Potter was asked
by a physician to help him determine whether he
could follow his patient's wishes and stop blood
transfusions, knowing the patient would then die.
The 72-year-old patient had been receiving almost
continual blood transfusions for two months as a
treatment for her fatal form of hemolytic anemia,
blood disease.

Judge Potter was "torn by the dilemma," a
reporter wrote. The patient's treatment "seemed
as bad as the disease."(41) His solution to the
dilemma:

"I can't decide whether she should
live or die; that's up to God," said
the judge. But, he added, "a person
has a right not to suffer pain. A
person has the right to live or die
in dignity." With a somewhat calculated
indirection, he therefore ruled that
Mrs. Martinez could not be forced to
accept any treatment that was painful.(42)

The transfusions, which had been prolonging death,
were stopped, and one day after the Court's
decision, the patient died.(43)

In two Wisconsin cases in the Probate Division
of the County Court for Milwaukee County,(44)
Judge Michael T. Sullivan denied a request for

permission to operate on an elderly woman who was
facing certain death and had already undergone two
operations, and also denied a requested order for
blood transfusions to be given to a 41-year-old
woman, a Jehovah's Witness, who was comatose and
who, prior to becoming comatose and with the
approval of her family, had rejected such transfusions. In fact, in this latter case, the patient
had previously signed a release form, refusing
consent for the transfusions and releasing the
hospital from any liability. Judge Sullivan explained his actions (the cases were not reported)
in a very lawyer-like article in a law journal.(45)
He cites many rules but reveals no personal feelings, although he does endorse a right to die.

Perhaps the most meaningful example both of
judicial ambivalence in cases involving the right
to die and of the burdens which can be placed on
a judge deciding such a case may be seen in the
case of Karen Ann Quinlan.(46) The trial judge in
Morristown, N. J., who presided at the Quinlan
proceedings, Judge Robert Muir, Jr., could hardly
have been prepared for this experience by his prior
four years of judicial service, or by his legal
experience in the law of municipalities, his
speciality prior to being appointed to the
Superior Court in 1971.

One group of citizens, opposed both to discon-
tinuing any medical treatments for Ms. Quinlan and
to allowing courts to get involved in what they
viewed as purely medical decisions, argued
vigorously that it would be playing God to stop
medical life support systems assisting Ms. Quinlan.

Theologian Martin Marty was quoted on the
other side:

> When in any other age [Karen Quinlan]
> would be dead, then I believe that it
> is not playing God to stop extraordinary
> treatment. In fact, it is playing God
> to keep her alive. (47)

This talk of "playing God" did not impress Judge
Muir, who is an elder of the Presbyterian Church
in surburban Mendham, N. J. (48) Conscious of the
unique role in which he found himself, he seemed
anxious to emphasize both his sense of humility and

his lack of identification with deities of any variety.

The Quinlan case admittedly involved some unusually emotional aspects; institutional religious values were also explicitly in question. The Quinlan family came into court accompanied by their parish priest, Father Thomas J. Trapasso, and with the public support of their bishop. Testimony centered, in part, on Joseph and Julia Quinlan's religious beliefs, and in that connection, a Papal Allocutio of November 24, 1957, was introduced in evidence at the proceedings. (49) It is an address entitled "The Prolongation of Life," which was delivered by Pope Pius XII to a group of anesthesiologists in which he emphasizes that there is no obligation to use extraordinary means to prolong life.

Early in the hearing, one of the Quinlan family's lawyers, James Crowley, sought to present testimony from a Catholic theologian of the status of the Papal statement and on other aspects of Catholic doctrine on the sanctity of life. In responding to the objections of the other attorneys to such testimony, Crowley sought to justify such testimony by saying that the witness could testify about the "weight" to be given to the Papal Allocutio. When Judge Muir asked Crowley what he meant by "weight," the lawyer responded: "Is it fallible? Is it not infallible? Where this document comes from the Pope, as it does, where does it fit in within the framework of this man's [Joseph Quinlan's] individual decision?" (50) Judge Muir, quite taken aback, looked at Crowley and said, almost unbelievingly: "Are you suggesting that I have to get into the question of Papal infallibility?" (51) Then recovering his composure, he ruled that such matters were irrelevant and that the testimony of the witness was unnecessary and would not be heard.

As if the posing of such weighty theological issues were not enough, the capacity of Judge Muir (or any judge) to deal with the issues presented by the Quinlan case was questioned bluntly during the closing arguments of the lawyers. Ralph Porzio, the lawyer for Ms. Quinlan's doctors, who opposed the family request to discontinue the respirator, first wondered aloud

whether such decisions were not more properly
left to doctors and not judges.   After conceding
the medical condition of Ms. Quinlan, the difficulty of defining death, and the anguish which the
Quinlan family had undergone, Porzio asked (and
answered by implication) this rhetorical question:

> Now does all of this, your Honor, justify
> this Court's intervention to mandate the
> steps to terminate her life?   And here
> there are seemingly great complexities
> that involve ethics and morality and
> theology and law and medicine and
> sociology.   And many other fields.   But
> what can the law do....there are some
> limitations as to what the law can do to
> resolve some human problems. (52)

After then outlining a number of situations
in which he noted that "the Law" could not eliminate pain nor bring back life, (53) Porzio went
on to the "playing God" theme as he contemplated
the Court's weighing the issues and ultimately
defining the quality of life:

> I have said at the outset that there are
> many degrees or graduations of quality
> of life, and once that becomes the
> determining factor, then I have to say
> this: You [referring to Judge Muir]
> make a God-like decision... To use as a
> measuring rod the quality of life in
> determing life or death calls for
> titanic decision-making.... (54)

Two weeks later, on November 10, 1975, Judge
Muir issued his written opinion in this case.   Few
judges have exposed the pain and anguish of the
decision-making process as did the judge in this
case.   Obviously disturbed by the implication of
Porzio's allegation that he might be "playing
God," Judge Muir, after describing the facts and
legal issues involved, went on:

> I pause to note the scope of my role.
> I am concerned only with the facts of
> this case and the issues presented by
> them.   It is not my function to render
> any advisory opinion.   In this age of
> advanced medical science the prolongation

of life and organ transplants, it is
not my intent nor can it be, to resolve
the extensive civil and criminal legal
dilemmas engendered. (55)

Having made this formal statement in his best
judicial manner, he then uttered a truly unusual
cri de coeur:

It is suggested to make "the life or
death" decision here involves apotheosis
and should therefore be avoided entirely.
It is the nature of the judicial process,
once set in motion, to deal with an issue
no matter how grave its consequences. To
carry out the judicial process, I most
humbly suggest is NOT [capitalized in the
original text] an effort to exercise
Divine Powers.
   The onus of the judicial process for
me, in this instance, is unparalleled. (56)

We can hardly expect any greater candor than this
from a jurist presiding over a hearing conducted in
a fishbowl setting, from which every nuance was
reported daily across the world.

Chief Justice Richard J. Hughes, writing from
the more Olympian heights of the New Jersey
Supreme Court, exhibited no such emotion over his
later evaluation of this case as had the earlier
judge. Speaking for a unanimous Court, Judge
Hughes, in a 59-page opinion, (57) praised the
efforts of Judge Muir, stated that he was correct
in declining to authorize the withdrawal of Karen
Quinlan's respirator "under the law as it then
stood," (58) and then proceeded to change New
Jersey law so as to make such withdrawal legally
possible.

Our earlier review of selected judicial decisions has revealed the difficulties which some
judges have felt in making the difficult choices
involved. Of course, these difficulties are not
peculiar to judges only; a great many conflicting
interests are almost inevitably involved in a
decision to terminate medical care:

The problem is not only of government
interests versus individual rights, but

the state's interest in preserving
and protecting life seems to mandate
continuation of care. The interests
of the patient's family and friends
conflict; that they suffer anguishing
financial and psychological burdens
points to termination of care, yet
their strong feelings of love, loyalty
and hope point to continuation of care.
Finally, the patient's own interests
conflict: though the value of continued
existence is incalculable, the patient
might have an even greater interest in
choosing a minimum quality of life. (59)

One might argue that the ambivalence of judges
as exhibited in right to die cases in no way
differs from a similar sense of conflict found in
these situations with physicians, the patient, and
relatives of the patient. Yet, there do appear to
be important differences. The judge is not trained to make the medical decisions in such cases;
further, he or she will not be involved in the
actual termination of life-sustaining procedures,
if such a decision is ultimately reached. Judges
often resent, as did Justice Markowitz, that they
are being asked to make what they believe should
be medical, not legal, decisions. The fact that
physicians come to courts with such requests out
of their fear of civil or criminal liability if
they make these decisions without judicial consultation and blessing does not make the judicial task
in these cases any simpler.

Also, judges are neither as emotionally involved with the patient as are relatives or
friends, nor can they feel the pain or fear of
suffering often experienced by the patient. The
judge is an impersonal, more objective observer
of the scene; this is the very reason why he or
she is felt to be more capable of making such
decisions rationally while balancing all of the
interests and values involved. Judges, however,
are people who are just as uncomfortable with
issues of death and dying as are their neighbors.
They have, but don't always discuss, their own
feelings about such matters, and as Judge Muir
in the Quinlan case demonstrated, the role of
decision-maker in such cases can be a very emotion-
wracked one.

Yet the judge is distinctively the arbiter of legal authority, the principal representative of the State whom the public consults. Obviously, the judge is neither being consulted for medical expertise nor for an ability to compassionately relate to the patient's plight. The role of the judge is to provide a legal imprimatur on behalf of the State to the physician or to the family of the patient. Yes, the doctor may discontinue use of the respirator. No, the surgeon may not operate on this patient. Judges seem to be ambivalent in the dispensing of this authority on a case-by-case basis.

Perhaps one way to relieve judges of this dilemma is to let other representatives of the State make such decisions. Indeed, the argument has been made that legislatures can balance these interests in a much better way than courts and are more suitably equipped to do so; and that while the New Jersey Supreme Court's opinion in the Quinlan case

> may have been an eminently moral and
> practical effort to render justice,
> its lack of sound precedential
> principles concretely illustrates the
> limitations of the judicial approach. (60)

This view proceeds on three assumptions: [1] that legislatures have the power to make laws which can provide immunity from civil or criminal liability for decisions made by physicians, family or even the patient; [2] that the legislature is in a position to take a more adequate reading both of public opinion and of expert opinion than a court which cannot hold public hearings; and [3] that the legislature can "provide a framework within which courts can better decide the merits of each particular case" and can inform individuals of their rights and the procedures to be followed in implementing them. (61)

My own inclination would be to support all three of these assumptions. Yet recent experience suggests that legislators are as ambivalent on these issues as are judges, and that they are not anxious to seize the initiative. Early in the proceedings in the Quinlan case, Attorney General William F. Hyland suggested to Judge Muir that any

change in legal precedent which would allow Mr.
Quinlan the authority he was seeking should not
come from a court decision, but from legislation.
He said that he anticipated legislation on the
issue because "the [New Jersey] Legislature had
failed to come to grips with the problem." (62)
New Jersey Governor Brendan T. Byrne announced two
days later that, under certain circumstances, he
was prepared to support legislation authorizing the
withdrawal of life-sustaining medical procedures
from terminally ill patients. While he was not
prepared to recommend specific legislation,
Governor Byrne stated his belief that "the broad
public interest in the Quinlan case would inspire
legislative action." (63) This turned out to be
overly optimistic. Several days later, the only
physician in the New Jersey Legislature, Joseph
McGahn, said that he did not foresee a legislative
solution to the legal problems posed by the Quinlan
case. Dr. McGahn said that the Legislature would
not be able to "decide on the constititional definition of life" and that "the courts would have to
lead the way in cases such as the Quinlan case."
(64) Thus, the responsibility was thrown back to
the courts where, in fact, the decision was
ultimately made. (65)

The only legislative success thus far in passing a law to deal with right to die cases occurred
in California where the Natural Death Act (66) was
signed into law by Governor Edmund G. Brown, Jr.
This statute which attempts to protect physicians
who discontinue medical treatment of terminally
ill patients went through nine revisions on its
legislative journey prior to passage, and the resulting tangle of compromises and restrictions has
left no one happy with the resulting statutory
language. Yet, the California legislators are not
interested for the moment in further attempts to
clarify the Acts, as the wounds from last year's
battles have yet to heal.

Even if legislators were less reluctant to
take a clear stand, courts would inevitably be
involved in the consideration of such issues.
Either one of the parties concerned will seek to
establish its position by judicial fiat, or the
courts will be asked to interpret uncertainties
in the language of the applicable legislation.
Thus, it seems that one cannot avoid, even if one

would prefer to do so, the involvement of courts
and judges in future cases involving termination of
medical care.

If this premise is correct, then we can at
least seek to alleviate the difficulty which
judges often appear to find in passing judgment on
these issues. Because they are not prepared by
their law school training or their professional
experience as lawyers and judges to deal effectively with these issues or even basically to compre-
hend their magnitude and complexity, they should
be helped to become aware of these issues before
they have to face the making of a judicial decision
requiring their thorough mastery. Thus, I wish to
make a modest proposal. An interdisciplinary and
cross-professional effort should be initiated by
lawyers, physicians, ethicists, theologians and
other relevant professionals to design a program
which could introduce the consideration of these
problems to trial and appellate judges. These
sessions could provide concrete information, a
chance for judges to begin examining their own
feelings about death and having to make decisions
involving life and death, and an opportunity to
hear from judges who have already faced such
challenges. Judge Muir, Justice Markowitz and
Judge Sullivan could undoubtedly give some helpful
advice at this point.

Arrangements for such "continuing judicial
education" could perhaps be made with the coopera-
tion and support of the National Conference of
State Trial Judges and the Appellate Judges'
Conference, both of which are affiliated with the
American Bar Association. To be successful in my
judgment, however, the program would have to be
interdisciplinary in order that judges would learn
from professional experiences and insights other
than those of their own colleagues.

As Justices Hugo Black and Benjamin Cardozo
have pointed out, judges come equipped with all
the human limitations and assets. Ambivalence
on the part of judges and legislators in dealing
with "right to die" questions is no more surpris-
ing, therefore, than similar reactions on the part
of physicians, patients, and their families. But
if we are going to continue to seek the assistance
of judges in making or validating decisions in

this area, then we have an obligation, I believe, to be equally concerned with the distinctive human and professional needs of those men and women whom we ask to make these decisions.

FOOTNOTES

1. U. S. Supreme Court Justice Hugo L. Black
    dissenting in Green v. U.S., 356 U.S. 165,
    198 (1958).

2. John T. Noonan, Jr., Persons and Masks of
    the Law (New York: Farrar, Straus and
    Giroux, 1976), p. 15.

3. Circuit Judge Warren Burger dissenting in
    Application of President and Directors of
    Georgetown College, Inc., 331 F.2d 1010,
    1017 (D. C. Cir. 1964); Justice Jacob
    Markowitz in Petition of Nemser, 51 Misc.
    2d 616, 624, 273 N.Y.S.2d 624, 631 (Sup.
    Ct. 1966).

4. New Haven: Yale University Press, 1921.

5. Ibid., p. 141.   (Emphasis added.)

6. Ibid., p. 168.

7. William W. Winslade, "Ambivalence"
    (unpublished paper), p. 1. Significant
    portions of this paper are incorporated
    in a forthcoming article by Dr. Winslade on
    the California Natural Death Act which is
    scheduled to appear in Volume 26, Issue No. 4
    (Summer 1977) of the De Paul Law Review.

8. Ibid., p. 3.

9. Edwin S. Shneidman, Deaths of Man (Baltimore:
    Penguin Books, Inc., 1974), p. 81.

10. Ibid., p. 82.

11. Winslade, "Ambivalence," p. 3.

12. Lon L. Fuller, The Problems of
    Jurisprudence (Brooklyn: The Foundation
    Press, 1949), p. 2.

13. Ibid., p. 10.

14.   Application of the President and Directors
of Georgetown College, Inc., 331 F.2d
1000 (D.C. Cir. 1964).

15.   Ibid., pp. 1006-07.

16.   Ibid., p. 1004.

17.   Ibid., pp. 1009-10.

18.   Application of President and Directors of
Georgetown College, Inc., <u>supra</u> note 3.

19.   Ibid., p. 1017.

20.   Ibid., p. 1018.

21.   Ibid.

22.   U. S. v. George, 239 Fed. Supp. 752
(D.C.D. Conn. 1965).

23.   Ibid., p. 754.

24.   In the Matter of Powell v. Columbian
Presbyterian Medical Center, 49 Misc.
2d 215, 267 N.Y.S.2d 450 (Sup. Ct. 1965).

25.   Ibid. at p. 215, 267 N.Y.S.2d at pp. 450-51.

26.   Ibid. at p. 215, 267 N.Y.S.2d at p. 451.

27.   Ibid.

28.   Ibid.

29.   Ibid. at p. 216, 267 N.Y.S.2d at p. 452.

30.   Collins v. Davis, 44 Misc.2d 622, 254 N.Y.S.
2d 666 (Sup. Ct. 1964).

31.   Petition of Nemser, <u>supra</u> note 3.

32.   Ibid. at p. 617, 273 N.Y.S.2d at p. 625.

33.   Ibid. at p. 618, 273 N.Y.S.2d at p. 627.

34.   Ibid. at pp. 619-20, 273 N.Y.S.2d at p. 627.

35.   Ibid.at p. 620, 273 N.Y.S.2d at p. 628.

36.   Ibid. at p. 621, 273 N.Y.S.2d at p. 629.

37.   Ibid. at pp. 622-23, 273 N.Y.S.2d at p. 630.

38.   Ibid. at p. 623, 273 N.Y.S.2d at p. 631.

39.   Ibid. at p. 624, 273 N.Y.S.2d at p. 631.

40.   Ibid. at p. 624, 273 N.Y.S.2d at pp. 631-32.

41.   TIME, July 19, 1971, at p. 44.

42.   Ibid.

43.   Ibid. The official title of this unreported
       case is Palm Springs Gen. Hospital v.
       Martinez, case No. 71-12678, Circuit Court
       of Dade County, Florida, decided on July
       2, 1971.

44.   Guardianship of Gertrude Raasch, No. 455-996,
       decided January 25, 1972; and Guardianship
       of Delores Phelps, No. 459-207, decided
       July 11, 1972.

45.   Michael T. Sullivan, "The Dying Person -
       His Plight and His Right," New England Law
       Law Review (Spring 1973), 8:197-216.

46.   This case began on September 12, 1975 as
       Docket No. C-210-75 in the Chancery Division
       of the Superior Court of Morristown, Morris
       County, New Jersey. The official title is
       In the Matter of Karen Quinlan, An Alleged
       Incompetent.

47.   TIME, Oct. 27, 1975, p. 41.

48.   New York Times, Oct. 23, 1975, p. 43, col. 3.

49.   Exhibit DD-2, Record, Vol. 3, p. 435 (Oct.
       22, 1975).

50.   Record, Vol. 3, p. 462 (Oct. 22, 1975).

51.   Ibid. at pp. 462-63.

52.   Record, Vol. 5, pp. 663-64 (Oct. 27, 1975).

53.   Ibid. at pp. 665-66.

54.   Ibid. at p. 675.

55.   Matter of Quinlan, 137 N.J. Super. 227,
       252, 348 A.2d 801, 815 (1975).

56.   Ibid. at ftn. 5, p. 253, 348 A.2d at p. 815.

57.   Matter of Quinlan, 70 N.J. 10, 355 A.2d
       647 (1975).

58.   Ibid. at p. 45, 355 A.2d at p. 666.

59.   Note, "The Tragic Choice: Termination of
       Care for Patients in a Permanent Vegetative
       State," New York University Law Review (May
       1976), 51:285-310; see p. 296.

60.   Ibid. at p. 297.

61.   Ibid. at pp. 297-98. See the proposed
       statute at pp. 298-306.

62.   New York Times, Sept. 23, 1975, p. 79, col. 3.

63.   New York Times, Sept. 25, 1975, p. 1, col 6.

64.   New York Times, Oct. 1, 1975, p. 49, col. 3.

65.   The New Jersey State Senate Committee on
       Institutions, Health and Welfare held
       a one-day hearing on January 26, 1977 to
       consider among other bills, Senate Bill
       S-1751 by Senator Anne Martindell. This
       Bill provides for the signing of a document
       to discontinue "maintenance medical treat-
       ment" if the signer becomes terminally ill.
       It is patterned after a bill prepared by
       the Society for the Right to Die in New
       York City.

66.   Calif. Health and Safety Code, Secs.
       7185 et. seq.